THE BEST OF

DENTAL HUMOR

THE BEST OF

DENTAL HUMOR

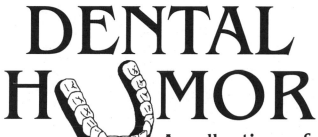

A collection of
articles, essays,
poetry, and cartoons
published in the
dental literature

COMPILED AND EDITED BY

STEPHEN T. SONIS, DMD, DMSc

PROFESSOR AND CHAIRMAN
DEPARTMENT OF ORAL MEDICINE AND DIAGNOSTIC SCIENCES
HARVARD SCHOOL OF DENTAL MEDICINE
CHIEF, DIVISION OF ORAL MEDICINE,
ORAL AND MAXILLOFACIAL SURGERY, AND DENTISTRY
BRIGHAM AND WOMEN'S HOSPITAL
BOSTON, MASSACHUSETTS

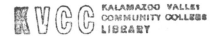
HANLEY & BELFUS, INC.
PHILADELPHIA

Publisher: HANLEY & BELFUS
             210 S. 13th Street
             Philadelphia, PA 19107
             215-546-7293
             Fax 215-790-9330

North American and worldwide sales and distribution:

       MOSBY
       11830 Westline Industrial Drive
       St. Louis, MO 63146

In Canada: Times Mirror Professional Publishing, Ltd.
             130 Flaska Drive
             Markham, Ontario L6G 1B8
             Canada

The Best of Dental Humor   ISBN 1-56053-067-7

Library of Congress Catalog Card Number 96-36809

Last digit is the print number: 9 8 7 6 5 4 3 2 1

DEDICATION

For my brother, friend and colleague, Andrew L. Sonis, D.M.D.,
who continues to be my greatest inspiration for the subject of this book.

CONTENTS

THE VIEW FROM THE CHAIR: PATIENTS' THOUGHTS

LESSONS IN PRACTICE MANAGEMENT

ODE TO A DENTAL HYGIENIST (AND A FEW OTHERS)

CONTENTS

LIFE BEYOND THE OPERATORY

TALES OF DENTAL EDUCATION

DISEASE, PATHOLOGY, AND RESEARCH
(AND OTHER THINGS IN JOURNALS)

CONTENTS

DENTISTRY, THE LAW, AND REGULATION

DENTAL HISTORY AND DENTISTRY PAST

BITS AND PIECES

INTRODUCTION

About three years ago, an editor at Hanley and Belfus asked if I would be interested in editing a book on dental humor. Hanley and Belfus had already had successful publications on medical and nursing humor and felt that there was both material and interest for such a work in dentistry. I had just completed editing a couple of academic books and thought that a humor book might provide some comic relief. While I love the clinical, research and educational aspects of dentistry, I have always found room for humor in what we do. The task didn't sound too ominous. After all, it seemed that there were always humorous articles and cartoons relating to dentistry in virtually every magazine or journal I picked up. Every issue of the *New Yorker* seemed to contain at least a couple of dental cartoons. However, as I started work on this book, I found I could apply the "there's never a cop around when you want one" rule to material.

Being used to conventional forms of research, I started my search for material by first querying the 9,232,103 references in the databases of the National Library of Medicine. I was pleased to find that articles on dental humor and wit constituted 0.00055% (n = 51) of the database. A printout revealed such classic titles as *Dentistry and the nineteenth century American humorists, An investigation into the relationship between human beings and Norfolk terriers* and *Psychische Gesichtspunkte fur Zahnarzt und Patient bei Ausbleiben des erwarteten Behandlungserfolges [Pyschological considerations for the dentist and patient in failure of expected result of treatment].* More contemporary titles included *Latexhibition: using humor and creativity as HIV/AIDS prevention tools in a university setting* and *Pfaff vermenschlichte die Zahnheilkunde.* Needless to say I was inspired.

Since it was clear that Medline was not the treasure trove I hoped, the search for dental humor was extended to journals not included in the database and to lay publications. As you might imagine, this required an enormous amount of work, much more than I could have accomplished on my own. Consequently, I was very fortunate to have assistance from our clinical research coordinators, Kerry Costello, Jennifer Thompson, Jamie Geier and Aparna Mekala, who in addition to their routine duties, spent many hours in Countway Library poring through journals in search of dental humor and corresponding with authors for permission to reprint pieces. One database was not enough, and neither was one library. The staff of the University of Pennsylvania Dental Library are thanked for allowing access to their collection and for chasing addresses and miscellaneous other items.

Mike Bokulich, the publisher's editor for this book, worked with me throughout the project. Without his expertise, guidance, and hard work, this book would not have been completed. He could always find additional pieces, find an elusive author, and keep the book moving when we thought we were at a dead end. Linda Belfus, who has the patience of Job, has again been a pleasure to work with. Finally, I would like to thank my best friend, advisor and wife, Trudy, who helped with many aspects of this work from researching jokes to proofreading and editing.

We hope readers will conclude that dental humor is not an oxymoron.

Stephen T. Sonis, D.M.D., D.M.Sc.

CONTENTS

ART AND THE ART OF DENTISTRY

Dentistry has long been a fruitful subject for almost every art form. Paintings, poems, plays, movies, novels, cartoons, and even music have featured our profession. From *McTeague* to *Little Shop of Horrors* to the Three Stooges, dental humor—some of it on the dark side—has permeated art. Who doubts that *Marathon Man* is on the mind of many patients as they contemplate endodontics on a maxillary central incisor?

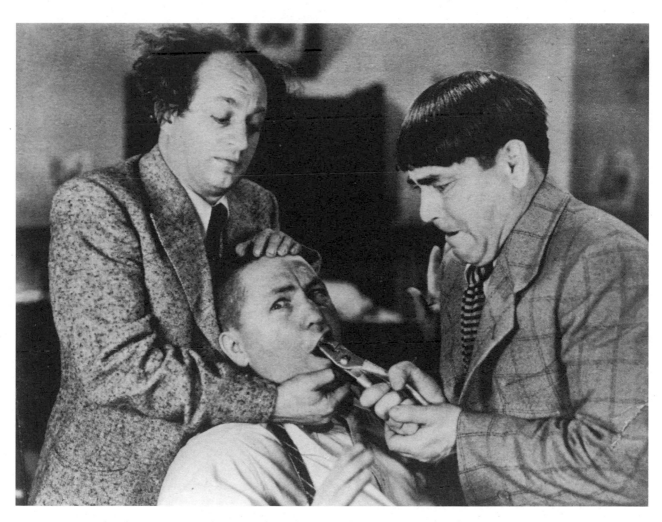

The Three Stooges. Healthy, Wealthy, and Dumb, 1938. With permission of Photofest, New York.

LOCK LIPS—MONKEYSHINES
IN THE BRIDGEWORK*

S.J. Perelman

I can pinpoint it unerringly—it was the last week in June when I became conscious of a faint but unmistakable emphasis on dentistry in the press, almost as if someone were giving me a sly nudge. Nothing explicit, to be sure—just a line here and a paragraph there that, along with an incisor that wobbled when I bit into piecrust, honed my sensitivity to the subject. The first hint, a mere throwaway in a Broadway gossip column of the *News*, concerned a well-known thrush: "Lois Hunt, who sings with Earl Wrightson, is a licensed Pennsylvania dentist." The item might have packed more journalistic punch, I felt, had it portrayed her as unlicensed, but, as a resident of the state and longtime admirer of the lady, I glowed at the diversity of her achievements. Shortly afterward another and more obvious dental innuendo caught my eye—an orthodontic coup in the Midwest reported by the *Times*. "False 'talking' teeth have been developed," it stated, "to tell a University of Michigan dental researcher what it feels like to chew.... This is the first time single teeth capable of radioing information have been made. The teeth are designated to disclose the forces that act on them when they chew.... The talking teeth resemble ordinary false teeth used in bridgework. Each tooth is packed with six miniature radio transistors, twenty-eight electronic components, two rechargeable batteries, and an antenna."

Psychosomatic or not, by Thursday of that week the slightest pressure on my incisor caused it to sway like a Lombardy poplar, and, bowing to the inevitable, I phoned my dentist in the county seat for an appointment. Dr. Crunch, his receptionist divulged, had flown to Malaya to seek gutta-percha for fillings, but he had left as locum tenens a Dr. Fangl, who would see me forthwith. As it happened, I had some policies to discuss in Doylestown with Bodley Risk, my insurance man at Gollancz-

Durnheim, Inc. ("Our Motto: Gol-Durn Your Problems"), and after the fine print had been spelled out to my consternation, I went along to Crunch's office. A jet-haired Juno with smoldering eyes, in a surgical tunic that accentuated a notable physique, welcomed me into the inner cubicle and, enveloping me in the scent of Mitsouko, secured a plastic bib around my neck. Supposing the vision to be a new nurse, I asked when Dr. Fangl would materialize.

"Oh, forgive me," she said, in a husky contralto that awoke memories of Kay Francis, Elinor Glyn, and tiger-skin couches. "I'm Bianca Fangl—I thought perhaps you recognized me. I sang with Lloyd Pettibone."

"Not *the* Bianca Fangl?" I asked incredulous. "The one that does all those operettas and record albums?" Her lashes fluttered acknowledgment of my homage. "I've enjoyed you for years. Your renditions that is," I corrected hastily.

Her smile revealed three hitherto invisible dimples. "Why, how sweet of you," she murmured. And how perceptive of her to notice my sweetness, I thought with thumping heart. "Yes, Lloyd and I just closed at the Whisper Lounge in Detroit, and I always sandwich in a few weeks' dental practice during layoffs. All this bending and stretching"—she illustrated—"it's good for the figure, I think."

"Wizard," I concurred. "Your colleague—is he a part-time dentist too?"

"No, Lloyd's in a slate quarry up in Lehigh County," she replied. "He drills those shingles they use on roofs." The similarity of avocation reminded her of professional duties, and she reached briskly for a dental mirror. "Now, what seems to be the trouble?"

The problem was crystal clear, the solution even more so. The errant tooth would have to be replaced with an artificial one cabled to its neighbors.

The principle, as Dr. Fangl expounded it in terms comprehensible to a layman, was the same as that used in stabilizing a snow fence or the spiles of a wharf. I retreated into a network of evasion: whatever shakiness she had observed was pure nervous reflex, I was psychologically unprepared for any drastic measures, and, furthermore, my underwriters disclaimed all responsibility should I conk out under anesthesia. Dr. Fangl pooh-poohed my qualms. The changeover could be effected painlessly in an hour, thanks to technological advances. I was in superb physical condition, she said, with an admiring squeeze of my biceps—virile enough for a man twice my age. Goose that I was, I knew I was succumbing to feminine witchery, but some indefinable fear—perhaps that if I remained obdurate she might try to kiss me into submission—eroded my will, and I weakly gave in.

The actuality, happily, was less rigorous than I anticipated. True, there were moments when Bianca's *embonpoint* heaved with exertion and my fortitude was threatened, but forty minutes later I was able to view the new incisor, anchored firmly in place, in a hand mirror. As she smoothed my wayward toupee and I relaxed, she favored me with a few selections from her repertoire that skillfully implemented the Novocain—"Cherry Pink and Apple Blossom White," "Three Little Fishies," and "How Much Is That Doggie in the Window?" Then, as I rose to leave, she issued a word of warning.

"This restoration I've done is something new," she said. "It's very complex and terribly sensitive to its environment."

"You mean it hates being where it is?" I asked, affronted.

"Goodness, no," she said quickly. "You've got a lovely mouth, I assure you." The impulse to swap tributes was alluring, but I mastered it. "The idea is, you must be awfully careful of the things you chew. We've got ways of finding out."

"Who—you and that Lloyd Pettibone?" I asked, with a surge of jealousy.

"Never mind, foolish boy," she said. "Just stay away from pretzels, hard rolls, apples, and such, and don't crack any nuts with it. Now, run along, and remember, Big Sister's watching you."

So vivid was the impact Bianca had made on me, and so earnest her injunction, that I took pains to screen every morsel I ate the following week. On Sunday morning, however, there occurred the first of a chain of incidents that shook me profoundly. Deep in Suzy Knickerbocker's log of the activities of Stavros Niarchos, the Alfred Strelsins, and Contessa Pecci-Blunt, I was munching half a bagel larded with Novy and cream cheese when the phone rang. The rich contralto purr over the wire belonged to only one dentist on earth, and behind it I could hear the sound of water splashing on a tiled surface.

"It's Bianca—Doctor Fangl," she was saying urgently. "I just stepped out of the shower to get your message." Whether it was the bagel or the image of my caller in her birthday suit that constricted my speech, I replied thickly that nothing was amiss, I hadn't called. "I *know* that," she said, impatient. "I got a flash from your jaw. You misbehaved—you're eating a bagel."

"I—I just had a couple of bites," I stammered. "It wasn't toasted, honest. . . . Look, hadn't you better slip into a fleecy robe or something? You're liable to catch cold."

"Now, don't shilly-shally." Her tone became that of a schoolmistress. "I cautioned you to avoid stress on that tooth, and I expect cooperation. Soft buns, corn bread, Danish, or scones, but that's it—do you hear? You're lucky you've got a guardian angel in your head to look after you."

My own interpretation, requiring no dental diploma, was that I was harboring a spy, and though I yielded with a show of grace, my appetite began to dwindle appreciably. After a fortnight of yogurt, semolina, junket, and similar pap, I was so undernourished I burst into tears over trifles and even turned faint during commercials for dog food. The breaking point came one evening as I was passing a Fanny Farmer shop in the Port Authority Bus Terminal. Dizzied by the heavy aroma of chocolate, I ran in, bought half a pound of fondants and marzipan, and then, swept away, added a piece of butterscotch to nibble while my purchase was being wrapped. I had barely swallowed it before a saleswoman emerged from the stockroom with word of an imperative toll call from a Dr. Fangl in Pennsylvania.

Dumbfounded at the extent of her surveillance, and hot with resentment, I sprang to the phone. "See here, Doctor, what is this?" I demanded. "Can't a person raise his sugar curve without you poking your nose in? I'm entitled to *some* privacy!"

"And so am I," she retorted, with equal heat.

"Where do you think I was when I got that alert just now? For your information, I was in a porch hammock with a very attractive gentleman of my acquaintance."

I apologized for interrupting her tête-à-tête, observing rather waspishly that Lloyd Pettibone's dialogue was clearly more fascinating than any I could offer.

"None of your affair who it is," she said, and I realized in an access of misery that some Doylestown square had checkmated us both. "The issue now is that you deliberately and willfully ignored my orders. You're playing with fire, gnawing on a confection like that. What do you suppose I put in there—an emery wheel?"

"I can't help it," I whimpered, striving to excite her compassion, if nothing else. "I'm run-down, famished. I need an incentive to go on living—the feeling that someone like you cares—"

"But I do, Sidney," she assured me, with sudden warmth. "Most dental sessions are humdrum, but ours was—well, different. And besides, I'm constantly in touch with you, as you know. Now, we'll overlook this slip for once, but hereafter, anytime you're worried about some goody—be it apples, caramel, licorice, whatever—promise to check with me beforehand. Cross your heart."

Well, I acceded out of *force majeure,* and, I suppose, the same quenchless hope that impelled Hillary to vanquish Everest. Nothing untoward happened until I was confronted with an ear of corn several weeks later at a dinner party. My host, a novice in the country, flaunting his first produce, was hungry for approbation; it was unthinkable to plead I must have clearance from my dentist, and I plunged ahead. The humiliation that followed was insupportable, beyond description. Even though Bianca's jeremiad was not audible to the company, my own reaction was, since the phone was but a few yards distant from them. Unable to endure her scorn, I gave her the full weight of my tongue. I impugned her dental skill, branded her a heartless flirt, and, distractedly reaching for the ultimate insult, accused her of singing off key. The rest of the evening was a nightmare. The other guests, many of whom were in wine, were quick to seize on and embroider my outburst, and I was subjected to raillery so merciless that I sickened. In the circumstances, there was only one anodyne. I poured myself a thimbleful of brandy, and at two o'clock was conveyed home in the rear of a neighbor's jeep spread out like a starfish.

It was the measure of a deeply generous nature that when Bianca entered her office the next morning and beheld me in the chair, haggard with remorse, not a word of censure did she utter. Instead, and with a sad gentleness that shamed me afresh, she subjected her handiwork to a painstaking scrutiny to insure it was intact. Then, signifying I was dismissed, she turned away—the better, I suspected, to hide the moisture dimming her great, lustrous orbs. Some gesture of penitence, some avowal of my regard other than the check I would mail her in a few months, was obligatory, and I forced myself to make it.

"This . . . this is the end, I suppose," I said, sighing. She nodded, but made no reply. "Bianca, I know I've been a beast. Still, it wasn't all my fault, believe me. It's your tooth that came between us—this little white sneak, blabbing everything I did. Oh, I realize I'm not the only pebble on the beach—you must have scads of other patients with talking dentures to worry about—but let me say one thing. You're straight, and clean, and fine, and you deserve a man who can fulfill the best in you."

"Oh, my very dear." Suddenly she was all radiance again, my slight forgiven. "You're trumps, too, so I'll tell you a secret. Lloyd Pettibone and I are washed up. I've found a new partner here in Doylestown with a glorious voice—the fellow who runs the meat counter at Hutzler's Market. We've been rehearsing nights in my hammock, and we open a week from Tuesday at the Megrim Room in Newark. Guess who I want at a ringside table that night to sing to?"

Well, I was there, and I can testify she killed the people. Her partner was OK—if you go for that sort of schmalz, which I personally don't—but I think I deserve some credit also. I ate chow mein with soft noodles during her act so that my tooth wouldn't distract her, and, to judge from the melting looks she threw me, she got the message, all right. Your singing dentists like Bianca Fangl aren't made in a day. One has to keep on trying.

ADDRESS TO THE TOOTHACHE*

Robert Burns

Robert Burns' "Address to the Toothache" was first published in The Belfast News Letter *of September 11, 1797, over a year after the author's death on July 21, 1796, at the age of 37. Burns, Scotland's great poet, wrote the poem while he was tormented by a violent toothache. As Burns had been known to have strong and attractive teeth, the onset of oral troubles may be attributed in part to his then generally poor health, financial worries, and depletion of spirit. Burns wrote the "Address" in the dialect of a small province of his country, and the following glossary explains many of these words.—Ed.*

My curse upon your venom'd stang,[1]
That shoots my tortur'd gooms alang,
An' thro' my lug[2] gies monie a twang
   Wi' gnawing vengeance,
Tearing my nerves wi' bitter pang,
   Like racking engines!

A' down my beard the slavers trickle,
I throw the wee stools o'er the mickle,
While round the fire the giglets[3] keckle[4]
   To see me loup,[5]
An', raving mad, I wish a heckle[6]
   Were i' their doup![7]

When fevers burn, or ague freezes,
Rheumatics gnaw, or colic squeezes,
Our neebors sympathise to ease us
   Wi' pitying moan;
But thee!—thou hell o' a' diseases,
   They mock our groan!

Of a' the num'rous human dools[8]—
Ill-hairsts,[9] daft bargains, cutty-stools.[10]
Or worthy frien's laid i' the mools,[11]
   Sad sight to see!
The tricks o' knaves, or fash[12] o' fools—
   Thou bear'st the gree![13]

Whare'er that place be priests ca' Hell,
Whare a' the tones o' misery yell,
An' rankèd plagues their numbers tell
   In dreadfu' raw,[14]
Thou, Toothache, surely bear'st the bell
   Amang them a'!

O thou grim, mischief-making chiel,[15]
That gars[16] the notes o' discord squeel,
Till humankind aft dance a reel
   In gore a shoe-thick,
Gie a' the faes[17] o' Scotland's weal
   A towmond's[18] toothache.

[1]sting; [2]ear; [3]giggling youngsters; [4]cackle; [5]leap; [6]flax-comb; [7]buttocks; [8]woes; [9]harvests; [10]stools of repentance; [11]graves; [12]annoyance; [13]prize; [14]row; [15]fellow (the devil); [16]makes; [17]foes; [18]twelve months'.

A VISIT TO DR. RIGGS*

(With Apologies to Henry Wadsworth Longfellow)
Murray Schwartz

Dr. John Riggs is generally recognized as the first American periodontist, and for several decades in the 19th and early 20th centuries, periodontitis was known as Riggs disease. His wide reputation for successful treatment of the condition led Mark Twain to consult him after being referred by a dentist friend. Twain left an unpublished essay called "Happy Memories of the Dental Chair" in which he describes Riggs and his treatment in Twain's own special style. Since Riggs was so well known, perhaps other New England literary figures were also his patients. How might Longfellow have described a visit to Dr. Riggs?—Ed.

Listen, my children, and you shall hear
How Dr. Riggs treated my pyorrhea:
On the 18th of April in seventy-five,
A dentist friend said, "For your teeth to survive,
You'd better see Riggs; he can make your gums
   thrive."
He told my how Riggs had established his fame
By success with the ailment that now bore his
   name.

Riggs' office in Hartford, up one flight of stairs,
Was furnished quite simply; he put on no airs.
I seated myself, though my insides were grim,
And fearfully opened my molars to him.

He looked and he poked; he probed and he
   prodded,
And every so often his gray head, it nodded.
He said my disease was no uncommon thing.
It afflicted a pauper as much as a king.

He went on to explain, with increasing ardor,
How he must remove all my bad bone and tartar.
I cried, "Must that be? Is there no other way?"
With a gleam in his eye, Riggs proceeded to say:

"Some day there'll be methods and marvels
   galore,
And techniques that have never been thought of
   before;
Such as membranes put in with new surgical
   handcrafts,
And subepithelial soft tissue gum grafts.

"There'll be fibers that dentists will nudge into
   pockets,
So that very sick teeth can remain in their sockets.
There'll be fixtures that we will implant by the
   score,
As we look for locations to place even more.

"There'll be A-splints, and experts will show how
   to use them,
And bone grafts that work if we just won't abuse
   them."
Then the gleam died away and Riggs said with a
   smile,
"I'm afraid that those marvels must wait for a
   while."

He picked up a tool and he started to scrape,
While I looked around for some means of escape.
But his hand was quite steady; his stroke it was
   sure,
As his scaler moved swiftly, my problem to cure.

When finally through, he carefully told me
How to brush and to floss, but he never would
   scold me.
And for many years after, at least four times a
   year,
His skilled ministrations made one thing quite
   clear.

No matter what special techniques were in
   fashion,
Twas his regular recalls that kept my teeth
   gnashin'.
So each time I'm in Hartford I give a small cheer
For Dr. Riggs' treatment of my pyorrhea.

*Reprinted with permission from the *Journal of Periodontology,* 65(8):805, 1994.

EXTRA CREDIT*

Dr. Richard Galeone

Legend has it that I am descended from a hundred generations of goatherds. Men who flocked up and down the green hills of Apulia, consuming calories like locomotives. Men who squirted milk into the bottles and jugs of village women. Men who did whatever men did to make ricotta cheese. Men of the mountains, of the earth, of manual labor. But then, in the hundredth generation, Biagio, the Tarantine, escaped the poverty of the south, came to Pennsylvania and became a butcher. His son was my father. So how was it that a descendent of all these men of manual labor was unaccustomed to working with his hands? Well, I'll tell you. I don't know.

My parents, however, thought of education as an emancipation from manual labor. Use your brain. As children, the only thing we used our hands for was the turning of a page and various lusty pursuits which did not seem to advance artistic ability. Of course, I hadn't thought this through upon my arrival at dental school and, in any case, I am not convinced that the explanation would have altered Dr. Himmler's opinion. The man terrified me. This brought him pleasure.

Hooves would grow from my wrists as he approached, wax inlays exploded, denture wax-ups metamorphosed into candle drippings. Just the smell of his custom-blended parfum triggered catastrophe. On such occasions, he would smile broadly, revealing a row of cervical gold foils beneath a band of scurvied tissue and make an entry into his black book. It might have been his grocery list. I might have been G.V. Black.

"Ah, when I look at your vork, Galeone, you make me feel like a genius. Ever think of law school?" he sneered looking at the debris on my desk.

"Yeah, well," I quipped.

"Look at Goldberg's vork. Maybe you'll learn something."

Goldberg and several others tried to console me with pitying looks, exchanged knowing glances, and turned back to their work. They pulled away as if from a leper and shunned the sight of my hoofy hands sloughing off.

We all wondered about the white carvings in the glass cabinet that Dr. Himmler kept locked at the front of the room. Miniature animals, automobiles, and plant life were displayed on immaculate glass shelves—a tribute to the memory of dexterous students from the past.

"As a project," he announced one morning, "for extra credit, take a double bar of Ivory soap and carve something for me. I don't care what it is. Animal. Vegetable. Mineral. It can be anything you want but make it good. Due next Friday."

Extra credit, I thought. Voilà! I worked myself into a lather thinking about what I might carve. I considered a nude. Something I could really get into. But as it was a bar of Ivory soap I kept picturing myself in the shower with it and had to wash the idea from my mind. I came, finally, upon a delicate ceramic fawn resting on a corner shelf in the living room. It was the right size and shape. Its head was down, pulling at a clump of grass. Even the color was that of Ivory soap.

At first I worked feverishly. I imagined myself picking a slab of marble from a quarry wall in Carrara and shipping it to my studio. No one would see the masterpiece before its completion. It might take years, decades, eons—ah, life was short. Life was cruel. Soap shavings stuck to my desk, to my chair, to the floor around my desk. My mother wanted to know what the hell I was doing. But I held my tongue. They would be amazed, shocked! Whispers of "master" would be heard as I padded humbly by.

It was only after several days and the approach of the deadline that I realized one could not work soap to the delicacy of ceramic. My fawn, while grazing next to the ceramic, was thick and heavy. It looked the bumpkin next to the city slicker, a genetic defect of its cousin. It was only extra credit af-

*Reprinted with permission from the *Pennsylvania Dental Journal*, (Mar/Apr): 55–56, 1994.

ter all. It couldn't actually hurt my grade. I would get what I got. Very few whispers of "master," I realized, would tickle my ear.

On the morning of the unveiling, I gazed with horror at Goldberg's little white Ferrari. It glistened like mother-of-pearl in the morning light. Hand-buffed. Hard wax. I could smell the motor oil, hear the purr of the engine. The girl sitting next to the driver wore a very short skirt and had what appeared to be a perfect set of shade #62 ceramco crowns on her upper anteriors. Her hand was on his leg well above the knee. To my amazement the driver looked uncannily like a smiling Dr. Himmler.

Say lavee. I would pick up an application to law school on the way home. I was so depressed that my caloric intake dropped below 5,000 calories at dinner, and I lay awake all night wondering how my family would react to news of my career change. Whispers of "I told you so" already ricocheted about my room in preparation for the fateful announcement. I pictured Aunt Gessupina shaking her head sadly as she walked off into the garden to pick some oregano. I saw myself applying for work at the glue factory, eating baloney sandwiches from a lunch pail. When I finally fell into a fitful sleep, I dreamt that Dr. Himmler stopped round to purchase a vat of glue. When I saw him, my hands turned to hooves that my boss tried to cut off over a pot of boiling glue.

In the morning Goldberg punched me in the arm.
"You're a sly one," he said.
"What do you mean?"
"You're kidding," he said.
"No."
"You didn't see the cabinet?"
"No."

I looked up and there it was: my sculpture on display among Himmler's menagerie. The professor was walking toward me with a smile. Was this some joke? Some further humiliation? Were these hands too inept even for law school?

"Good vork, Galeone. That's the finest buffalo I've ever seen. I can tell you put a lot of time into it."
"Thank you, professor. I guess I just got lucky."
"Nonsense."

"O THAT THIS TOO SOLID FLESH SHOULD MELT..."*

The Dental Secrets Of Shakespeare's Characters

Marc Tyler

Until recently, one of the better kept secrets in the academic world of university scholars was the fact that Professor Reginald Q. Cuttlefish, of Oxford, foremost authority on William Shakespeare, was a graduate of the Warwickshire School of Dentistry. Now, in his latest book, "The Secret Lives of Shakespeare's Characters," Professor Cuttlefish's extensive knowledge of dentistry has surfaced. In a special chapter called, Special Chapter, the professor informs us that William Shakespeare, the illustrious bard of Avon, was plagued with dental woes throughout his life and that his preoccupation with the oral cavity is revealed through his characters. Thanks to Professor Cuttlefish's research, we are now able to gain a better insight into the many characters Shakespeare presented, especially their dental problems.

Why did Cassius have a "lean and hungry look?" On the surface it would appear that this was the result of his anxiety in plotting the death of Caesar, right? Wrong! According to Professor Cuttlefish, Cassius was wearing a new set of immediate dentures and was so busy with his treacherous scheming that he never had the time to return to the dentist for an adjustment. As a result, he was in constant pain and could hardly eat and had lost eight pounds the week of the Ides of March. Who wouldn't have a lean and hungry look? Some scholars ask, "Why didn't he leave out his dentures?" The answer is academic. Without dentures, nobody would have understood a word he said and the whole play would have bombed.

When Lady Macbeth cries, "Out, out, damned spot!" we are all led to believe that she is referring to the blood stains on her clothing. This is true, but only in part. Actually, there is a two-fold meaning here. Though not written in the play, we know that Lady Macbeth was in the bathroom trying to wash the blood from her hands and clothes after the foul murder. While there, she looked into the mirror (an opportunity no woman passes up, especially one as vain as Lady Macbeth) and couldn't help but notice the large discoloration on her upper right central incisor. With her husband dead and on the prowl for a new lover, she was understandably distressed by the ugly spot. If she wasn't on stage so often she might have had time to see the royal dentist and had it corrected—but that's show business.

In *Hamlet*, Act I, Scene 5, Horatio, speaking about Hamlet, says, "He waxes desperate with imagination." This is an obvious reference to Hamlet's incipient periodontal condition. Beset with innumerable problems, the Dane's gingival condition had worsened and he was trying desperately to remove the plaque with waxed dental floss. However, if he had cut some of his speeches short he may have found the time to visit his periodontist and we all would have been better off. Yet, Hamlet was not so unaware of the need for regular check-ups and good dental care as one might believe. For in Act III, Scene 2, he says to his mother, "No, good mother, here's metal more attractive." She had been wearing an ill-fitting acrylic partial, and the young Dane, appreciating the value of a good cast metal appliance, is trying to persuade her to have a new partial made. But the Queen isn't listening to anyone who talks to ghosts, would you?

In *Richard III*, Richard the Duke of York says, in Act II, Scene 4, "Twas full two years ere I could get a tooth." Who is he kidding? Granted there weren't too many dentists in England at the time and that

*Reprinted with permission from *Tic* (Sep): 7, 16, 1987.

ART AND THE ART OF DENTISTRY

they were all busy—do you mean to say they couldn't find time to squeeze in the King's son? Or maybe he used to break his appointments and none of the dentists wanted any part of him. Professor Cuttlefish doesn't answer this question satisfactorily but he makes reference to the fact that the Duke always complained of headaches on the days when there was a boar hunt, so we are led to believe that Richard was just plain chicken.

There are many dental references in most of the plays. For example, Falstaff, suffering from food impaction, speaks about having his "pocket picked," and Worcester, in *King Henry IV*, says he is concerned about the "fear of swallowing," since he probably is suffering from an impacted wisdom tooth. There are also some blatant contradictions, for in *Cymbeline* we learn that the character believes that, "He that sleeps feels not the toothache," while Othello says, "Being troubled with a raging tooth, I cannot sleep."

Professor Cuttlefish says that in *Much Ado About Nothing*, there is indeed a conversation that is not only much ado about nothing but just plain stupid. In Act III when Benedick says, "I have a toothache," Don Pedro's advice is, "Draw it." To quote Cuttlefish, "Even if Benedick was a gifted artist how would a drawing of the situation remedy the problem?" We agree, and thank Professor Cuttlefish for presenting yet another facet of Shakespeare's characters. For those interested, the book can be purchased at Ye Olde Book Shoppe on Shonery Road in Stratford-upon-Avon.

LEAVE 'EM LAUGHING*

Laurel & Hardy

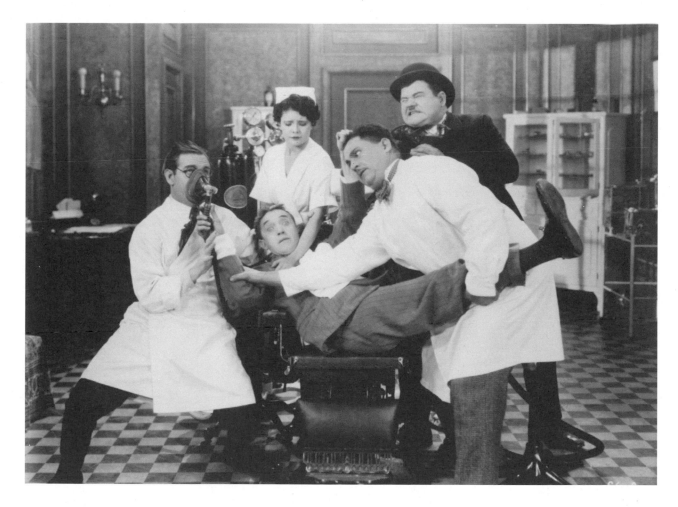

Stan, an "anxious" patient, has a toothache. With Jack V. Lloyd, Viola Richard, and Otto Fries.

*Leave em Laughing, 1928, Hal Roach/MGM Studios; with permission of Photofest, New York.

THE DAILY ROUTINE
OF PRACTICE

A survey completed by my classmates at the start of dental school concluded that the overwhelming majority of us chose dentistry as a profession because of the opportunity to "help people." (I should mention that "making artful objects" was also high on the list.) Few of us probably had any real clue as to the complexity of practice or the logistics of delivering care to patients. The routine of practice combines all the elements of a healthcare delivery system with those of a small, or in some cases not-so-small, business. Consequently, the daily practice produces a mixture of satisfaction, angst, and humor. And some days simply defy the label "routine."

SLEEPLESS IN LANSDALE*

Dr. Richard Galeone

Just as surely as darkness is the absence of light, misery is the absence of sleep's sweet balm. Aroused in the night by a great thirst, consequent to the intemperate consumption of a Nino's double-anchovy large, I groped toward the oasis of the bathroom and, not wanting to wake my wife, did not switch on the light.

In the dark I turned on the cold-water tap, filled the glass and lifted it to my dusty lips. But instead of cool water I was shocked to have a large insect enter my mouth and run back and forth from left to right at a terrified pace. Horrified, I spit the thing into the sink and turned on the light. A large black roach raced around the web of cracked porcelain at the bottom of the bowl. Tearing the roll of toilet tissue from the wall, I punched at the monster and missed. I punched again. I missed again. Clearly the brute's synaptic ability was greater than mine for when I swiped at him a third time, not only did he easily avoid my thrust, but he escaped down the drain with athletic agility. Denying this affront, I seized the hot-water spigot, turned it on full, and condemned my carapaced friend to a death by boiling water.

The knuckles of my right hand were bruised and bleeding and my vital signs danced capriciously as I sat down on the toilet seat to catch my breath. It was 3:33 A.M. and I had a full book of patients, including the fascinating Rodney Pike, scheduled for the next day. I abandoned, finally, any hope of falling back to sleep when I heard the first miserable chirpings of the birds.

As my disorientation and borderline psychosis were insufficient warning against the practice of dentistry, the episode at Gagger's Diner should have run up a red flag. It was eight in the morning but I was ready for lunch. I ordered a turkey club and sat at the U-shaped counter where one might see, at any hour, a gathering of introverts and assorted neurotics. A couple of people were hiding behind the *Daily News*, but the majority were simply staring into mugs of thick coffee. My cousin Crucifix was waitressing the counter that day and she brought me the sandwich. It was quartered and piled precariously with turkey, and each wedge was skewered with one of those long toothpicks with red cellophane party strips on the end.

After studying the geometry of the sandwich I determined to leave the toothpick in place, at least for the first bite, for control. But biting into the wedge caused it to rotate down so that the wooded spear of the toothpick gouged through the cortical plate of my chin and harpooned into the underlying cancellous bone. I believe I called out unprofessionally and threw down the sandwich, but the toothpick, with its little cellophane flag, remained behind, standing Excalibur-like in my chin at the head of a trickling stream of blood. Even the newspaper readers paused in wonder as I darted from my stool to the sanctuary of the men's room where I gingerly extracted the thing and soaked my chin in cold water. Crucifix wrapped the remains of the sandwich and, oblivious of this omen, I left for the office.

"Where were you?" demanded Lucretia, our receptionist, when I walked in. "Rodney Pike is locked in the patients' restroom and he won't come out. Mrs. Merryme wants to call 911. Wow, that must have been some zit on your chin."

"I cut myself shaving."

"Shaving? What, with a meat grinder?"

Terrific. My father wanted me to become a lawyer. But, no. I preferred to spend my life talking the mentally disturbed out of bathrooms. Rodney Pike was 42 years old and the dour-faced Mrs. Merryme, his case worker, was down on all fours yelling under the door.

"Rodney, if you're not out by the count of three you can forget about McDonald's."

"Come on, Rodney," I said. "It's only a little cavity. You're a big guy. You can do it."

"No."

Hey. Fine by me. I'll make like I actually want to

*Reprinted with permission from *Pennsylvania Dental Journal*, (Mar/Apr): 45–46, 1995.

contend with Rodney while I'm dizzy, nauseous, sleep-deprived and homicidal—for a minute or two —and then I'll give up. Visions of other careers careened about my mind: cataloguing beetle species in the Amazon; glacier photography in Denali; ambassador to France. Yes. Ambassador. Residence on the rue St. Sulpice, chauffeur-driven limousine, Armani suits, Valentino shirts. Ah, yes. Mr. Ambassador, Rodney won't come out of the bathroom.

Suddenly the door is thrust open and Rodney bursts forth totally naked—that's right, *nada*—and dashes around the waiting room amid the screams of Lucretia and Mrs. Merryme. Trying to remember my holds from Rodeo Dentistry class, I wrestle Rodney to the floor just as the door opens. It's Mrs. Lehman with her two daughters. I do not know what they thought at that moment as they beheld me lying on top of a naked man on the waiting room floor, but I'm fairly certain it did not involve referring friends and neighbors to our practice. Smiling like sheep, we hustled Rodney off to the operatory number one where we dressed him.

Rodney's eyes rolled in fear when he saw me pick up the anesthetic syringe, and his prehensile right shoulder shot up to cover his mouth. I tapped the plunger in order to embed the spear into the rubber stopper of the carpule of lidocaine. But guess what? There was no carpule in the syringe. So instead of embedding the aspirating tip into the rubber stopper, I again harpooned myself, impaling my thumb with the thing. Call me Ahab. I pulled. I twisted. I bled. But it did not withdraw. It would not come free. The only thing it would do was cause pain. Sharp, gnawing, wracking pain. Shaking, I wrapped my hand in a towel and flew down the stairs to the office of my friend and general surgeon, Jimmy Stone.

"What happened to your chin?" Jimmy asked.

"It's a zit."

"Wow. You better stay away from chocolate."

"Look, it's my thumb, not my chin," I said. "I got a syringe stuck in it. Thank God it was sterile."

"You're the one who should be sterile. You wouldn't want to pass this on."

He yanked out the syringe and altered my fingerprint with a couple of stitches. Then he wrapped my hand in gauze and I had my ticket home.

MURPHY'S LAW IN DENTISTRY*

Whatever Can Happen, Will Happen

Shelly Freisinger

There's many a practitioner out there who will agree with me that Murphy must have had dentistry in mind when he wrote his famous law: "Whatever *can* go wrong, *will* go wrong." I've been collecting tales, and I'm now convinced that Murphy, with his unfortunate law, holds a special place in his demented heart for the dental profession. I'll share some examples with you (as long as Murphy doesn't let my typewriter break, and the typesetters and printers don't go on strike).

First, there was the dentist who was working in an extremely busy welfare clinic. He had a child in one chair who was in need of having three teeth extracted from the upper left quadrant and three other teeth extracted from the upper right quadrant. The frantically busy dentist anesthetized one side of the arch and ran off to see several other patients. Five minutes later he returned, still feeling harassed by the busyness of his schedule, and proceeded to extract the teeth on the side of the arch that had not been anesthetized. The patient began squirming, and before long began screaming. The dentist had only completed one extraction before the patient was attempting to fight his way out of the chair. The dentist took the chart, and immediately noted that for future records, this patient should be considered "difficult to manage" and "a child with a very low pain threshold." That's one way of using a "problem-oriented" treatment approach.

While we're on the subject of children, the pediatric clinic recently suffered from Murphy's wrath. A 10-year-old boy, with a record of "fear of injection," was brought in by his mother for a restoration. His reluctance to be treated was made clear when it became necessary for the student and an assistant to bodily carry him from the waiting room into the operatory. He kept stalling, asking for water, asking to go to the bathroom, asking to speak to his mother. Finally, the student was able to complete the topical and local anesthetic and to insert the rubber dam . . . Again the child asked to go to the bathroom, and the student, exhausted and wishing he could wash his hands of this entire experience, consented. Out the boy went, past his mother in the waiting room and down the hall to the restroom . . . Twenty minutes passed . . . No child! The student, assistant, several instructors, and an anxious mother searched the halls of the school, the bathrooms, the cafeteria, and still came up empty-handed. The mother went home feeling extremely disturbed . . . Twenty minutes later she phoned to let the clinic staff know that her son had gone down the hall, past the bathroom, and out to a bus stop, where, using his fast-pass, he hopped on a bus and, rubber dam and all, said, "I've had enough dentistry for today, thank you."

Murphy strikes when least expected. Ask the endodonist who was examining a female patient with a lower first right molar that required root canal therapy. Now this woman, clad in a jumpsuit, was very attractive and had the body of a glamorous model. The endodontist tried to develop rapport with his patient. Upon close examination of the crowned tooth requiring treatment, he noted a rainbow baked into the enamel. The work was done with such precision that the dentist was taken aback and asked what gave her the idea to have this done to her crown. She proceeded to zip down her jumpsuit, exposing herself and revealing a rainbow tattoo in her cleavage. . . . The dentist, not wishing to blow his cool, continued the exam. To his surprise, the same molar on the lower left also had an image, a lightening bolt, baked into the enamel . . . He hesitatingly asked his patient what had given her the idea to have this done, and she proceeded to unzip her jumpsuit all the way down, now exposing a

*Reprinted with permission from *Contact Point*, 63(2):22–24, 1985.

lightening bolt that descended from below her navel . . . What would Murphy have written in this patient's treatment record?

Let's stick with Murphy's visits to endodonists for a while, as he seems to demonstrate a special interest in these specialists. There's the story of the dentist whose office is located on the 25th floor of a high rise building and who decided to try his own version of "The Towering Inferno" shortly after the release of that motion picture. He was treating a "high city official" who had a terrible quiver from Parkinson's disease. As we view the scene, this shaking patient is in the midst of root canal therapy. He is completely surrounded by the dentist, chair, dental unit and tray, and chairside assistant. It is difficult to discern whether he is quivering more from his condition or from anxiety due to the treatment.

Having completed the gutta percha insertion, the dentist asked his brand new dental assistant to pass him the alcohol lamp so he could sear off the excess gutta percha. Wanting to be helpful, the assistant turned the lamp upside down to ensure that there was plenty of alcohol in the burner, and in so doing, she spilled alcohol all over the lamp and onto the base of the chair. . . . The dentist lights the lamp, causing an explosion and setting his hand on fire. Seeing the explosion and his dentist's burning hand sets this poor patient into quivers that could be measured on the Richter scale. The dentist manages to maintain control and puts his hand into water . . .

Meanwhile, the base of the chair has caught on fire and the entrapped patient is beginning to see smoke rising. The dentist, still maintaining control, tells his assistant to run out and get a portable fire extinguisher. She panics and runs out into the main hallway in an attempt to get one of the high pressure water hoses. Time is passing and the fire is getting worse. The dentist yells for another assistant to get a fire extinguisher, and seeing the fire, this second assistant screams "fire" and runs out the door and down 25 flights of stairs. The dentist amazingly keeps his cool, gets an extinguisher himself, and puts out the fire. With things well under control, he now escorts his uncontrollably quivering patient out of the operatory and goes back in to open a window and let the smoke out. Unfortunately, the thick black smoke blows into the waiting room, and the remaining patients panic and run out . . .

There was this dentist who had a patient who was an artist. She was also a diagnosed schizophrenic who insisted that she could not be treated unless her psychiatrist was also present. The dentist happily consented. On the day of surgery, she insisted that the procedure be done while her head was held in the psychiatrist's lap. Again the dentist consented. The dentist did the procedure with the patient's head in the lap of her psychiatrist, who at the same time continuously massaged her temples. Several weeks later the artist presented her dentist with a painting of her recollection of the treatment experience. The rendering displayed two hands reaching into a chest and pulling out all of the organs . . .

Murphy has also been known to leave a lasting impression. . . . One dentist tells of the time when he had a lunch date with a new girlfriend. He inserted an impression tray in a patient's upper arch, and before he returned to complete his work, his attractive lunchdate arrived. Two hours later he returned to his office only to find several panicked assistants who had been trying everything imaginable in an effort to help the patient remove the solidly entrenched impression tray. . . .

If you've ever worried about the peer review process, you'll be happy to know Murphy's been there too. One doctor tells of the time he was on the peer-review committee, when a patient came in complaining of a dentist who had "cut my throat and made me look older." In fact, the dentist had been doing a crown preparation, and he had inserted a gingival retraction cord. She had spit the cord out in the sink and thought he had cut her throat. (Don't ask me how she jumped to that conclusion . . . Remember, Murphy's at work here.) She picked up the cord and later put it in her purse as evidence. She wanted the peer-review committee to approve her getting plastic surgery done, because the procedure had made her look older. As additional evidence, she brought in two passport photos, taken 5 years apart, to show that she looked older. The committee assured her that in 5 years she might indeed look older. However she would not believe the cause was anything but the dental treatment.

The peer-review doctor later asked her if she could get a copy of her radiographs. She brought them to this reviewing dentist, and he informed her that he would need to have them duplicated. Several days later she turned up at his office, accompanied by four policemen. She was doing a lot of screaming, and the dentist asked one of the officers why they were there. He responded that she had come into the police station with bizarre complaints, and they thought she was insane, so they were investigating. They removed her from the dentist's office, and he later learned that she had written to the governor of California about this same issue. With Murphy on the case, this one may reach the Supreme Court.

Denture patients often seem to be accompanied by Murphy. One dentist tells of his early experience as a graduating dental student in a midwestern dental school. He had to get a full upper and lower denture tried in a patient to fulfill his graduation requirements. Between the try-in visit and the final insertion the patient unfortunately passed away. He called the patient's children and convinced them that the patient would look much nicer buried in her full dentures and that he would be willing to pay for the entire treatment fee, if they would let him put in the denture.

One of the student's fraternity brothers was a relatively new clinical instructor, and this instructor drove along with the student to the parlor. There the denture was inserted in the patient, the instructor checked it off, and the student was able to graduate and ultimately become a specialist . . .

Orthodontists have been known to have run-ins with Murphy as well. There's the story of the recent graduate from an orthodontic program who was donating his services to a hospital clinic. Taking his first cephalometric head film on his own, he put the ear rods in the patient, took the radiograph, stepped back and removed the cephalometer from the ear openings, and the patient's ear came off. . . The child apparently had been born with a congenitally missing ear and was wearing a well-disguised prosthesis. Not exactly the best way to begin an orthodontic career.

Murphy loves to play tricks on dental students . . . like the guy who did an anesthetic on every single tooth in a patient's mouth, because he thought that was necessary before doing a full mouth x-ray . . .

Then there was the story of the Italian dental student who liked to talk expressively while waving his hands. He was in the midst of one such conversation in the school clinic, waving his hands wildly while holding an anesthetic syringe and needle in his hand. A fellow student was walking by, and as our friend was gesticulating, he waved his hand way out to the right and jabbed the needle into the fellow student's thigh. The victim walked about four more steps and went right down, his leg having been totally anesthetized . . .

One dentist tells of the time he was a student in oral surgery and saw something squirting down by his shoes. He thought someone was playing around with the water syringe. He looked again, and again there was the squirting liquid hitting his shoes. He looked up and saw a classmate with his anesthetic needle coming right out through the cheek of a patient.

Finally, there's the story of the dentist who *(Editor's note: Unfortunately, the rest of this article was erased from the word processor, and we have been unable to find any notes on the interviews that were taken to make this article possible . . .)*

MY PATIENTS ARE...

Campbell's Kids*
Martha Campbell

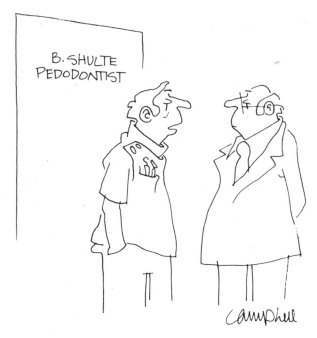

"My patients are a small but vocal group."

CLOSE TO HOME*

John McPherson

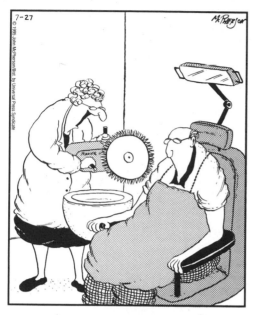

"OK, now, Mr. Weston. Let's start by taking care of that tartar build-up."

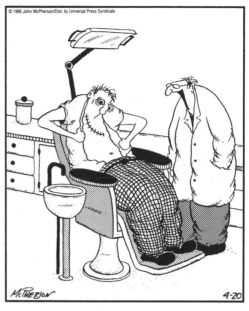

"That wisdom tooth on the right side was giving me a tough time. So I had to get at it from a different angle."

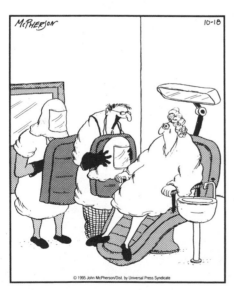

"Calm down, Mrs. Nursteen. There's nothing to be alarmed about. This is just some protective gear to shield us from any bits and pieces that might happen to be whizzing around the room during your root canal."

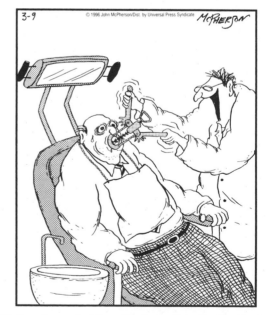

"Believe it or not, this particular tooth-extracting device was designed by a guy who makes corkscrews."

THE DAILY ROUTINE OF PRACTICE

YOU CAN FORGET THAT GAS!*

Michel R. Sturm, D.D.S.

While doing research for a roast to be used in the program at the IDA President's Dinner Dance, I called the chief's receptionist asking her to share a humorous or "fun story" from the office. "We don't get paid to have fun here," she replied.

That's not true though, is it? "A good laugh is the best medicine," it has been said, "even if you're not sick." It is almost impossible to smile on the outside and not feel better on the inside. Smiles, after all, are our business.

"Dentists are often driven to extraction."

Once upon a time, in the days before OSHA, AIDS, rubber gloves, and surgical masks, a well-intended Isaac Knapp oral surgeon proceeded with a routine tooth removal. His new assistant, Diane, was wide-eyed with wonder. Positioning the cold steel on an infected maxillary anterior tooth he gave a mighty squeeze. The tooth flew out of the patient's oral cavity, straightway into Diane's gaping mouth.

"A man with a sense of humor doesn't make jokes out of life; he merely recognizes the ones that are there."

Pediatric dentist Dr. Stainless Steel Crown was at dinner with friends. "How do you handle the unruly ones?" they asked. This Hoosier dentist described the hand-over-nose/mouth technique, explaining that this was usually very effective in calming the patient. "That explains it then," the mom added. "When we left your office last time, Bobby said: 'That Dr. Crown is nice, but I bet he kills a lot of little kids.'"

"There is hope for any man who can look in a mirror and laugh at what he sees."

A general dentist from West Central tells the story of a middle-aged woman who came into his office with a broken denture in her hand, wrapped in Kleenex. As she spoke to the receptionist, she curled her lips tightly and asked if the doc fixed dentures. She explained that she had broken hers and needed them badly since she had no spares. The receptionist asked about the dentures she had in her mouth at the moment. "Why . . . these are my husband's teeth. You don't think I'd go without teeth, surely!"

"Imagination was given to a man to compensate for what he is not, and a sense of humor to console him for what he is."

Dr. Malprop, a young practitioner from Isaac Knapp, gave a mandibular block to a nice-looking, generously endowed young lady and went on to the next room while it took effect. After a few minutes, Dr. Malprop returned saying, "Are your nips lumb?"

"Some people can't wait until April 1st to make fools of themselves."

The dentist was finishing up his last patient before lunch as the hygienist stuck her head in the operatory, saying that her patient was ready for an exam. Having lunch plans of her own, the hygienist then went on her way. The doctor finished the procedure and dismissed his patient. Forgetting about the lady in the other room, he deadbolted the office door and went on to lunch. An hour and a half later, he returned to a very unhappy hygiene patient.

*Reprinted with permission from the *Indiana Dental Association Journal*, 72(4):31–32, 1993.

"Laughter is like changing a baby's diaper—it doesn't permanently solve anything, but it makes life more acceptable for a while."

On Tuesdays, Fort Wayne's northside dentists like to gather at the Gas House Restaurant to "fix prices and tell lies." After lunch, one dentist bummed a ride back to the office with a fellow denticle. When he finished up that evening, he discovered his car missing. He called the police and reported it stolen. The officers soon arrived at the scene and asked where the car was parked when he last saw it. After a careful moment of soul searching, he replied "at the Gas House."

"If any man calls you a fool, don't insist on his proving it. He might do it."

One Indiana oral surgeon remembers a middle-of-the-night phone call from a patient whose toothache wouldn't wait. "Meet me at the office in 15 minutes," he replied. When he arrived, he found a young lady scantily clad in a revealing nightie. He prudently insisted that her husband accompany them during the procedure.

Many years later, the same dentist received another call and removed a tooth under similar circumstances. "If I'm not mistaken, you have been here before," he said. "That's right," she replied. "If I'm not mistaken," the suspecting surgeon added, "you were dressed in the same manner." The woman commented, "That's also right." The surgeon recalled, "And if I'm not mistaken, you never paid me for that procedure." Her husband then said, "That's correct. And you probably won't get paid this time either!"

"Everybody is liable to make mistakes but fools practice them."

An Indiana dentist recalls a second-year dental student with limited patient exposure who was assigned to her office in the extramural program. As the student assisted with an operative procedure, the dentist asked for a rinse. The student shot a stream of water up the elderly patient's nose. She sputtered and swallowed. The student was mortified and was very reluctant to do any further rinsing. At the next appropriate time, the dentist asked the student to rinse again, following the adage of getting back on the horse that threw you. The patient sat up. "Wait, wait!" She pinched her nose and added, "Okay, you can rinse now."

"Blessed is the man who can laugh at himself, for he will never cease to be amused."

She was a self-contained woman, not haughty, but confident. Her hair was well manicured, and her clothes were fashionable, but tailored. She was in for her first operative procedure with Dr. S. Mile, a new addition to the Fort Wayne dental community. "Relative analgesia" with nitrous oxide was a fairly new tool in dentistry in those days, limited, for the most part, to younger practitioners. It was a good promotional asset to a budding practice. "I would like to try the gas today, Doctor."

What the good doctor then meant to say went something like this: "Now sit back and relax. The nosepiece will just rest here over your nose. You are in control with nitrous, regulating its potency by breathing through your nose or alternately, with your mouth. Soon your fingers and toes will tingle and you will feel very relaxed." Instead, what he did say was: "Now sit back and relax. You are in control with nitrous. Breathe deeply and close your eyes and soon you will fart."

The young lady reached up, pulled off the nosepiece and was down the hall, almost out the door, before the good doctor could stop her to explain. "I don't know why I said that. I must have had other things on my mind. Please come back. Let me try again."

"Okay, Doctor. But you can forget that gas!"

HERMAN*

Jim Unger

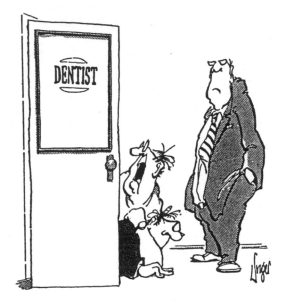

"Grab his legs!"

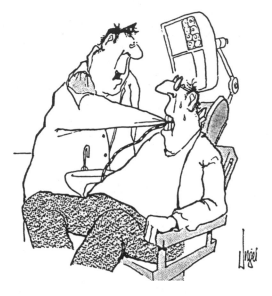

"I promise no more drilling if you let go."

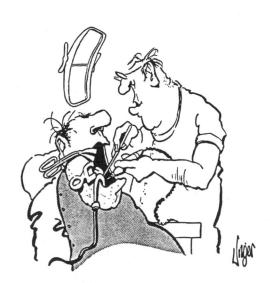

"Do you think the current economic policies will do anything to ease the overall unemployment picture and dampen inflation?"

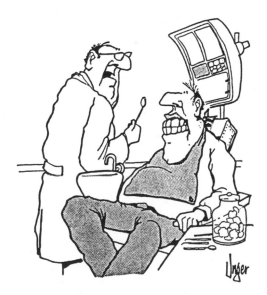

"It'll take you a couple of days to get used to them."

THE DAILY ROUTINE OF PRACTICE

VENTURE BEYOND BURNOUT: THE TIME IS NOW*

Robert E. Horseman, D.D.S.

You don't hear so much about burnout anymore. For a while there it was so common that the only people who claimed never to have experienced it to some degree were insensitive clods, individuals with exceptionally high tolerances to stress, or insensitive clods having exceptionally high tolerances to stress.

It got so that if you had a genuine case of burnout, it was tough finding a sympathetic audience. Dentists, as prone to burnout as the next mob, could usually count on each other for support, but it finally came to the point where burnout had about as much drama as the common cold, and you know how much sympathy you get for that.

To the rescue comes San Diego business psychologist Judith M. Bardwick, who has written a book entitled *The Plateauing Trap: How to Avoid It In Your Career and Life.*

If I read Bardwick correctly, "plateauing" is just what we've been looking for to replace burnout as the reason for the malaise and discontent we seem to fall heir to from time to time in our practices. Bardwick has it figured that there are three levels of plateaus:

- "Structurally" plateaued individuals have arrived at a stage in their careers where things seem to have stopped happening. Opportunity's knock is seldom, if ever, heard but more often is heard a discouraging word and the skies are more cloudy each day.

- Now if you have so mastered your techniques and procedures that you're getting bored out of your mind, you are said to be "content" plateaued.

- And, if your whole life seems to be bogged down with repetitive events and uninspired responsibilities, then you are labeled *plateaued in life.*

Not a pretty picture, is it?

Dentists and their staffs are particularly prone to plateauing. If this were not so, then all the practice management courses dealing with staff motivation, team efforts, productivity increases and the like would never attract enough participants to pay for the use of the hall, and the lecturers would be forced to seek some way to make an honest living.

Bardwick suggests that this plateauing often coincides with the onset of middle age, striking not only independent professionals, but housewives and business people alike.

Younger staff members, not yet confronted with mid-life, are leveled by low wages, lack of challenge, and absence of advancement, plus maybe bad complexions and a dearth of dates.

Bardwick argues that no one needs to be content plateaued. Employers should strive to enrich employees' work, presenting them with challenging assignments, etc.

Let's look at prophylaxis, a bread and butter procedure in most offices, one that has to be done day in and day out by either the dentist or the hygienist. Prophylaxis has been equated with doing the dishes by operators who have performed the task 5,000 or 10,000 times, but the dentist who does his own prophys is relatively lucky; he at least has other operations coming his way each day. The hygienist, bless her heart, faces a day, a week, a lifetime of prophys.

The Director of Dental Hygiene, addressing the freshman class, exults, "In 2 years, students, you will be scaling and polishing teeth for a living, educating patients in oral hygiene, and releasing the dentist to perform those tasks that only he can do. A noble pursuit." Thus, fired to almost religious fervor, the hygienist goes forth to rack up her first million prophys, only to fall victim to content plateau before she has finished the first 300,000.

In my office, I do all my own prophys, not that

*Reprinted with permission from *Dental Management,* 27(8): 18–19, 1987.

I'm too cheap to hire a hygienist, at least not entirely. It's just that I've discovered a way to make prophylaxis a challenging and rewarding experience, and I'd like to pass it along to other workers who may be asking themselves, "Is that like, you know, all there is?"

My Way

I had no sooner finished my 30th year in practice when I began to notice a certain ennui beginning to fall over me when I was in the midst of polishing a mouthful of teeth. At first I dismissed the feeling as a transitory anoxia resulting from the salad, cheeseburger with fries, and ice tea I customarily had for lunch, or the too-tight underwear that was a consequence of what I customarily had for lunch.

But on the occasion when I actually drifted into La-La Land over a patient, prophy angle slipping from my inert fingers, prophy cup dangling from my thumb, and nearly impaling myself on a scaler, I knew I had to seek a more challenging and exciting technique.

Here then, in all modesty, I present my breakthrough innovation:

Instead of starting with scaling the lower arch beginning with the lingual of the lower anteriors and then doing the lower left quadrant as had been my custom, then the lower right, followed by the same pattern in the upper arch and finally doing the polishing and flossing in the same sequence, I recklessly dared to pioneer.

It wasn't easy; pioneering seldom is. I broke into cold sweat, saturating a box of 4 × 4 wipes my concerned assistant kept applying to my forelock. Midway through, I was ready to call it quits, and only the determination to break the stranglehold that plateauing had on me kept me going.

Oh, the euphoria when I finished! My patient, sensing that history-in-the-making had just occurred, embraced me warmly. The entire staff gathered around, cheering and hoisting me onto their little shoulders, carried me off to the reception room for Dom Perignon and Ding-Dongs.

Let this be your credo, then, if you suspect you've arrived at a plateau. Strike out boldly where no man or woman has gone before. Dare to alter your established procedures and, like me, come to know the heady intoxication of having the guts to Take Charge of Your Life. Or, you might hire a hygienist.

JUST A THOUGHT*

Edward Samson, F.D.S.

People of the western world, the over-developed faces as distinct from the under-developed, lesser breeds without the law, have a deep hatred of teeth. "Teeth are a trouble coming, a trouble to keep, and trouble going." Almost ritualistically, they repeat that bewhiskered old platitude. Yet the same thing could be said of many another necessity—money, husbands and wives, life itself. Our teeth alone of all the body's organs and parts are objects of a profound and perpetual loathing and, by association, so is dentistry. Few people hate their stomachs, even ulcer-ridden ones. Not many nurse a grudge against the appendix, the liver and the colon, though these can be as untrustworthy as teeth. There is, as far as I know, no recorded case of renophobia. And how many persons can be discovered who obsessively dislike their gallbladders? There may be individuals, even small fanatical groups, who detest some area of their anatomy—pancreasphobes, or antitonsilists—but there is no such universal antipathy for these organs as there is against teeth among the civilized and privileged, the educated nations.

Psychologists can, no doubt, account for this; social biologists, ethnologists and any of the learned 'ologists who delight to explain us to ourselves would doubtless account for our tooth-hatred, at least to their own satisfaction. Whatever the likely cause, the effect is most distressing. Millions of *soi-distant* civilized people who wash themselves daily or weekly, never clean their teeth; some of them are quite pleasant folk one wouldn't mind asking in for bridge. In Great Britain only one house in ten owns a toothbrush. How many use it is not disclosed. As many others visit a dentist only to lose neglected teeth which have kept them awake by aching, either in their own jaws or their children's. There are, of course, a few reactionary old diehards who brush their teeth as assiduously as any "savage," attend the dentist regularly, and consider the loss of a tooth, as did our untutored forbears, to be a disgrace—people today as egregious as a stern father or, in remote places, a disciplined child. These are an exceptional minority. The rest of us prefer to be rid of our teeth, along with all the trying procedures necessary to keep them.

Radical But Sensible

The dental educationists, hoping against hope, and ever struggling to eradicate this ubiquitous tooth-loathing, try to disseminate a tooth tolerance, even a respect for teeth. While they pursue their work with missionary zeal, if small success, the rest of us frustrated dentists sometimes wonder, in our despair, whether it would not be easier, and more acceptable, to render the nation edentulous—universal, neonatal exodontia. A large proportion of our people, we are officially told, is already wholly or partially toothless by middle life so, why not anticipate the inevitable, save thousands of dentists their fruitless labors, the taxpayer millions of pounds, and remove all teeth from their crypts in all people at birth, or soon after? Most of the nation would be only too delighted; the Treasury would be ecstatic.

There would, we can be sure, be a few opponents to the scheme, there always are—an affront to the freedom of the individual; official and unwarranted interference with his liberty. Inevitably, too, a Society for the Protection of Natural Teeth would be formed; a late but welcome notion. That being so, total extraction need not be compulsory, but, like smallpox vaccination, voluntary but persuasive. The majority, however, would readily agree, if for no better reason than to escape forever the need for dental treatment. An eminent dental surgeon now removes wisdom teeth from their crypts in quite young children as a prophylactic measure, thus forestalling the many discomforts caused by these errant teeth and the later need of a trying,

*Reprinted with permission from the *British Dental Journal*, 132 (6):243–244, 1972.

surgical operation. Universal exodontia, government-sponsored, perhaps state-subsidized, is just an extension of this same, useful principle. Admittedly it presents minor difficulties. Growing children would require new dentures at regular intervals, at some cost to somebody; but no more so than replacing outgrown shoes or suits. At first there might be difficulty in obtaining approval to supply, through the National Health Service, a succession of dentures to developing infants, though it is not without precedent since some 3,000 children under 12 already have full dentures. Moreover, considering the food mostly consumed in this country, how little it requires, or receives, mastication, it would be no loss to them if the population were left edentulous. (Remember that old man everyone knows, who hasn't had a tooth for years and eats ham bones with his gums.) Certainly sweet sucking and lolly licking require no teeth.

Exodontia à la Mode

Aesthetically, or for social reasons, the scheme would be opposed, at least at the outset, but artfully designed propaganda, especially from the arbiters of fashion, would soon overcome opposition. Girls who will balance themselves on pencil-point heels, wear emerald green wigs, paint their eyes to appear like Mongols by Picasso, will as eagerly display coral pink gums instead of teeth; particularly if it were à la mode and Mayfair or Paris were doing it. Nor would the boys be any greater problem. A quick glance at their haircuts (or lack of them), their facial topiary, their shoes, will demonstrate how little prejudiced they are against the changes and grotesqueries of fashion. Just persuade one pop singer to moan his dirge from a toothless mouth and every young Beau Brummel in the country will rush to join the avant garde "Gummers." (There must be a name for them if the vogue is to catch on.) Indeed, in view of the deep loathing of teeth, my proposal presents no serious difficulties; tonsils, adenoids and other expendable organs, less hated than teeth, are lightly discarded with never a regret.

Vivat Britannia

This way, too, England might well lead the world again, become a virile and major power. We would hear no more of the diseases and disabilities which bad teeth cause, the lost manhours for which they are responsible. The health of the nation would rapidly improve beyond belief; England would stand where once she did, though toothless. The vast expenditure saved in the National Health Service would free money for some urgent purpose: more Polaris submarines, or relaying railway tracks. Dentists might, it is true, be disgruntled at first. Extracting teeth from infants and babies, making a few dentures for them as they grow up would hardly keep them occupied, nor satisfy the objectives of a noble profession, though they, like the public, would soon adapt themselves to the change. Healthier, happier and living longer they would readily accept a reduced income (a process to which they are rapidly being accustomed), though I am not sure that would be necessary. Since 120,000 children are born every day, not all of them in China or Russia, quite a few prophylactic extractions would be required of our 14,000 dentists, enough to keep them busy most of the week. If, as well, dentures were to be supplied, if only occasionally to eat the necessary and tougher protein foods, or for festive occasions, dentists could be usefully employed for the rest of their lives.

I do not propose to present a memorandum on the subject to the appropriate ministry, nor to disturb its minister by having questions asked in Parliament. Neither do I expect my plan to be readily adopted (certainly not promulgated) by my profession. Likely enough the National Pure Water Association will support it, if only to save the nation from fluoride poisoning. Whatever the outcome, I shoot my arrow into the air—that it may stick in someone's conscience.

PATIENTS

Patients provide us with a rich source of professional satisfaction and gratification. Improving their well-being is why we do what we do. However, they are sometimes an enigma and behave in ways that are unpredictable, at best. While all of our patients are individuals, it is reassuring to know that we all have the occasional difficult or quirky patient. You may even find descriptions of some of your patients in this section.

CAMPBELL'S KIDS*

Martha Campbell

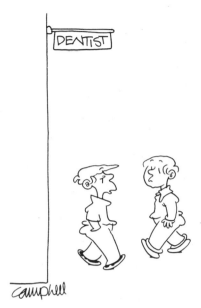

"Keep talking. He'll never hit a moving target."

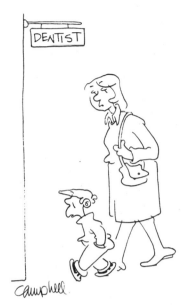

"Quit reciting the 23rd Psalm."

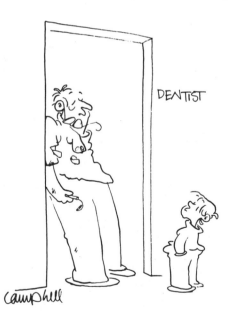

"Brush, kid. I can't stand a rematch."

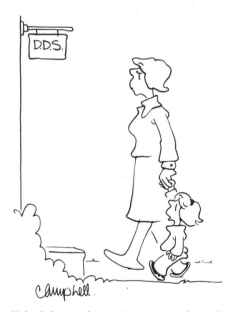

"I don't have to be carnivorous, you know."

LOCKJAW: A CASE STUDY*

Dr. J. John Portera

Dr. Portera has been collecting stories from fellow dentists for years and published his first set of them in Grinning & Grinding *(Best of Times, Inc., Pelham, AL, 1995). Volume II is underway.—Ed.*

Last weekend I was in Birmingham, attending a continuing education course sponsored by the University of Alabama. . . . [This] personal report of a case of lockjaw [was] reported to me by fellow attendant, Dr. Ricky Hess of Southside, Alabama.

According to Ricky, a patient appeared at his reception room window late one afternoon, unexpected, and obviously agitated by the look and sounds he was making. . . .

"Ah gotta see doc!" the patient said to the receptionist, his words coming through snarling lips and clenched teeth. . . . the vocal tone coming from deep in his throat, more like a dog's deep growl than the voice of a man whom she recognized quite readily.

"Why, James, what in the world is wrong with you?" the rather surprised receptionist asked.

"Ah can't git mah jaws open, dawg gonnit."

Before ol' James could attempt any more of an explanation, Dr. Ricky happened to pass by the receptionist area and, spotting his long time friend and patient, James, said:

"Hey, Jim. What's happening man?" Ricky, not aware of the exchange which had taken place just seconds earlier between James and his receptionist, was simply exchanging a quite common greeting between male acquaintances . . . though he knew, instinctively, Jim had to have some kind of dental problem. Our acquaintances, unfortunately, usually don't just drop by our offices for a friendly chat at 4 p.m. Yeah, Dr. Ricky knew something was amiss. . . .

"Ah needs yew, doc. Y'all gotta help me git mah mouf open!" Again, with tremendous strain, ol' James snarled out the guttural sounds which, even though spoken with a fine mist of spittle, were clear enough for Ricky to immediately motion for him to follow.

Ricky, like any conscientious dentist, personally seated his friend, and asked him to please open. . . .

"Darn, ah thawt ah told y'all . . . . ah can't open my jaws!!!" James, his face now blood red from the strain of trying to speak without opening his mouth, seemed on the verge of an anxiety attack and/or a manifestation of rabies . . . . by now, he was actually drooling saliva out the corners of his mouth.

Dr. Ricky, using a mouth mirror, couldn't really see what was keeping the patient's teeth clenched shut. He had just started to palpate James' muscles, to determine if they were in spasms, when the frustrated patient interrupted with. . . .

"It's super glue, yew fool. Mah teef is glued shut!!!" he said, with lips drawn back in a snarl-like look which, even under the pitiful circumstances, caused Ricky to think how much this man resembled a dog about to bite. He stifled, somehow, his urge to burst out laughing. . . . probably more out of fear of being attacked, than compassion.

Recognizing he had a very unique problem on hand, one he had not encountered in all his years of practicing dentistry, he calmly reassured the patient, and headed for the telephone. A call to a pharmacist he had great confidence in turned up a piece of advice which might, at first, seem quite unacceptable. . . . "Doc, you're going to have to use some acetone. Not much, just a drop or two at a time, until you loosen that stuff up. Just be real, real careful!"

Approximately forty-five minutes later, with dozens of cotton rolls and high speed evacuation being expertly handled by both dentist and assistant, the glue's strangle hold was finally broken on the teeth of one good ol' Alabama boy. Stuck on the palatal side of the upper left molar was the white

*Reprinted with permission from the *Mississippi Dental Association Journal*, 51(4):14, 1995.

nozzle from a tube of super glue. With this final obstacle being removed, Dr. Ricky asked a question any of us might have asked under similar circumstances:

"James, how in the heck did you get super glue in your mouth?" A question, quite reasonable and relevant but, under the circumstances, the frothing and frustrated patient didn't think was so innocuous. . . .

"Awraht, y'all thoo wif me?" the patient said, apparently angered and anxious to depart the dental office premises.

"Oh, James, we're not making fun, really. Heck, this could've happened to anybody," Ricky responded, realizing the patient was seriously embarrassed and needed a little reassurance that, whatever he'd done to get himself in the predicament, everything was going to be okay. Essentially,

he quickly let him know noone was about to have a seizure of laughter right in his face.

"Awraht, ah waz in my shop, fixin to glue a piece of plastic pipe. . . . y'all know how that thar nozzle spose to be cut awf or stuck wif a needle or sumpm sharp like that. . . . well, anyhow, the shawt of it is ah jus didn't wanna leave the shop to go git sumpm, so ah just bit the cap awf the darn thang. . . ."

Dental Moral: If you're in your own workshop, find yourself without the appropriate instrumentation for puncturing the nozzle of a tube of super glue and, in spite of this scholarly paper documenting the hazards of biting the nozzle off, you choose to make the same decision as good ol' boy, James . . . . please do not let your fingers apply any pressure to the tube, whatsoever, AS YOU BITE!!!

DIFFICULT DENTURE BIRDS*

Alex Koper, B.S., D.D.S.

Denture patients are "special" people because they have the problem of adapting to a prosthesis which affects one of the most sensitive and emotionally charged regions of the body. This must take place in full view of their friends, who, like baseball fans, are often opinionated and voluble "experts." The problem is compounded by the fact that in our North American culture, with its emphasis on youth, virility or femininity, and apparent immortality, the individual who lacks a normal and attractive dentition is disadvantaged. Therefore, it takes an uncommonly secure individual to accept dentures with equanimity.

During the time their dentures are being made, and later while they are learning to use them, our patients are dependent, frightened, "less than whole" people, and in many instances, regress to infantile behavior. There are individuals who have so much difficulty with their dentures that they never make an acceptable adjustment to them. Some wander from dentist to dentist in search of a solution to their dental needs, while others isolate themselves from society. These people are called *problem denture patients* or *difficult denture patients.*

Because American standards of function and appearance are so high, people whose physical or emotional limitations prevent adequate achievement with dentures suffer much and seek help from dentists. In other parts of the world where teeth are not looked upon as such a necessary and positive asset, these individuals might suffer little as a result of this deficiency. The difficult denture patient is, therefore, a more common problem to American dentistry, and is a product of our higher living conditions.

Identification of the Problem Denture Patient

Difficult denture patients have been described by Schultz[1] as "Individuals who present abnormal and uncommon denture problems. Because of the extreme complexities of their symptoms and their physical and emotional handicaps, these are difficult denture patients."

It is conceded that what may be an abnormal and uncommon denture problem for one dentist may be fairly routine to a more experienced practitioner. Also, the evaluation of the physical and emotional limitations a patient presents varies with the perception, observation, and experience of the dentist who treats him. It is also true that there are individuals who present severe challenges to all dentists who attempt to treat them. This poses the questions: "What makes a problem denture patient? Are there any criteria by which one may measure an edentulous patient in order to determine whether or not he is or will be 'difficult'?"

Some Characteristics of Problem Denture Patients

1. They complain.
2. They have pain.
3. They are hostile.
4. They exhibit regressive behavior.
5. They are tense, anxious, and appear unhappy.
6. They often have systemic illnesses.
7. They are inordinately preoccupied and conscious of their mouth and their dental problem.
8. They have an unrealistic fantasy regarding dentures.
9. They are often devious, deceptive, and disarming.
10. They are indefatigable and persevering in their efforts to obtain satisfaction.

While it may be true that some of these signs appear in patients needing types of treatment other than dentures, difficult denture patients exhibit all or

*Reprinted from the *Journal of Prosthetic Dentistry*, 17(6):532–539, 1967; with permission of Mosby, Inc.

most of these limitations, and often have additional handicaps which aggravate and intensify their symptoms.

Many edentulous patients become problem patients because they lack the physical apparatus to wear dentures successfully. Some are frustrated in their attempts to adapt themselves to a mechanical appliance which requires a rather high degree of neuromuscular skill and coordination. This most often comes at a time in their lives when they yearn for the comfort of familiar things and do not have the energy for this difficult task.

From Whistler's Mother to the Karate Hawk

Prosthodontic literature is replete with many analyses of these problems. There are certain individuals who cannot wear dentures successfully. Most writers on this subject attribute the causes for this lack of success to personality or emotional problems, physical problems, or failure of the dentist to provide the proper treatment for his patient. Whatever the cause of their lack of success with dentures, these people do not become problem denture patients unless they have had considerable experience as recipients of various kinds of dental therapy, and have thereby developed a particularly colorful and effective modus operandi which continuously and successfully thwarts efforts to construct workable oral prosthetic devices for them.

Only occasionally does one come upon discussions of denture failures in the literature.[2] Brewer[3] writes that he has no failures, just varying degrees of success. It might be erroneously surmised that the problem denture patient, the *Denturus Calamitous Americanus*, like the dodo bird and the silver dollar, is becoming extinct. Nothing could be farther from the truth. As yet, no statistics on the number and varieties of these birds are available, but informed observers estimate their number to be as high as 5 per cent of the denture-wearing population. Dentists who have encountered them are happy to disengage themselves from the clutches of these predatory creatures, and forget their experiences as quickly as possible.

Problem denture patients do not wear wrist bands that would identify them, and even well-trained veteran observers often fail to spot them. There simply is no *typical* problem denture patient. They come young and old, male and female, rich and poor. They may be as gentle and kind as Whistler's mother, or as aggressive as a politician a week before polling time. Generally, the female of the species is more colorful than the male.

Just as there is no stereotype of the problem denture patient, neither is there a uniform pattern to his behavior. Some of them will become unhappy and unmanageable at the first appointment; for others, the difficulties begin at the try-in appointment; while the majority wait until the dentures are completed before they begin their perverse maneuvers. Most of them need this time to measure their prey and plan their tactics.

I have been in a particularly strategic position to observe many exotic species of these Denture Birds. My experiences with grievance committees of the Los Angeles County Dental Society for the past 15 years, plus a practice which is quite heavily populated with many varieties of these creatures, has made an avid and wary Denture Bird watcher of me. Although I have never seen such rare specimens as the *Tawkorchoo Gobbler*, who uses two separate lower dentures—one for speaking and one for eating—I can readily identify five of the more colorful varieties which migrate from dentist to dentist in these United States.

Cookies, Sweet Talk, and Brass Knuckles

The most deadly is the *Karate Hawk*. He is a frequently observed predator whose insatiable need for new dentists to destroy compels him to fly in ever-widening circles. Forced by his reputation to seek out new and unsuspecting dentists to conquer, his hunting range is limited only by the amount of distance he can afford to travel. Most often discovered in the offices of recent graduates, this carnivorous species has a particular love for the flesh of new enthusiastic dentists who are full of knowledge and the confidence of youth. The female *Karate Hawk* is most difficult to identify because she is very deceptive. This bird successfully disarms her prey by continuous flattery and gifts of home-baked cookies.

Generally, she dresses conservatively, often refers to her activities as a devoted mother, her community achievements, and her pious dedication to home and husband. Concealed under a demure hair-do are two sharp horns, which are apparent only to the most wary observer. Hanging from her belt, and concealed in the folds of her clothing, are a pair of brass knuckles and a rubber truncheon.

One way to identify this hawk is to engage her in conversation about her previous dentists. It will then be observed that her eyes will turn fiery red, and her face becomes flushed as she relates her tales of conquest. Generally, this species wears an upper denture made by one dentist and a lower denture made elsewhere. In her purse she carries other trophies of previous kills. Another revealing clue is her handshake. This hawk, tiny and thin as she may be, can crush the hand of the average greeter. This is an important identifying sign, which I shall soon explain.

Generally, this species is very cooperative at the beginning of treatment, and will so lull the dentist that he will wonder why anyone with such excellent coordination and healthy ridges should ever have difficulty with artificial teeth. Only after the dentures are placed does the trouble begin. This patient has so much hostility, and is so strong, that she fractures porcelain denture teeth as though they were peanuts. After three days, all semblance of balance of the posterior teeth is destroyed, and the anterior teeth begin to crack away. If gold occlusal surfaces are used, the upper denture base soon splits under the stress of the extraordinary strength of this sweet, quiet-spoken, but deadly creature.

Going My Way?

The *Myway Magpie,* also known as the *Hertz Bird,* wears the feathers of a hard-working solid citizen whose occupation, if a male, might be an examiner for the Internal Revenue Service; the female is generally the president of the local chapter of the League of Women Voters.

The *Myway Magpie* generally appears with dentures worn in the pocket or purse. One hand holds a suitcase which contains a complete set of instruments for setting up teeth and waxing a denture base, in the other hand is a 25-year-old copy of Swenson's *Complete Dentures* (in a plain wrapper, of course), and coiled over one shoulder at a jaunty angle is a large whip of the type used by lion tamers.

At first an amiable creature, the *Hertz Bird* readily agrees to the fee and can hardly wait to get started. This is because having dentures made is an engrossing avocation for this bird, and the fee is rarely paid because the dentist seldom completes his treatment.

As its name implies, this bird must be "in the driver's seat." It should be pointed out that, at all times, this creature maintains a sporting attitude. In his conversations with the dentist, he will occasionally use phrases like "balanced occlusion" or "incisal clearance," and now and then he will chirp out the word "centric." If he does not feel he has given the dentist enough warning, he may casually mention the fact that he was a navy dental corpsman for three weeks during World War II.

The preliminaries are over when the try-in begins. Now the *Myway Magpie* takes charge of all aspects of the construction. No set-up is satisfactory. The teeth must be changed. Their color is wrong. They are too long or short, or they just do not feel right. Months may go by, and spouses or other supporting relatives may be called in to support the contention that a marriage is being ruined by the dentist's inability to achieve the proper esthetics for this person. Often, if the dentist lasts long enough, the patient will take over completely. The following is an excerpt from a grievance committee case; the dentist's reply to a patient's complaint. Here, in part, is the chronicle of his experiences with a *Myway Magpie:*

She threw her hands up in despair and said: "You just won't set them the way I tell you. If you will just give me an instrument I'll show you how I want them." I thought—"What have I to lose in humoring her? I've tried everything else without being able to satisfy her." So I lit the fire in the lab, set out a wax spatula and wax, and invited her to be my guest. I thought she meant to shift a tooth or two. That was where I was mistaken.

At 5 P.M., Mrs. B. was still setting teeth. Words cannot describe the results! "This," she said, "is the way I want them." I asked her repeatedly, "Mrs. B, are you sure that is what you want?" I asked her to assure me that she would be satisfied if we completed the case thus. She said that she would. That wax was a mess, to put it mildly. I assured her that we would not shift a tooth.

The completed denture was to be delivered on Monday . . . etc., etc.

It goes without saying that this patient won again, and was soon released by this dentist to fly to the next encounter.

Make Me Like I Never Was

The *Minewere Mallard*, also known as the *"I Usta" Duck* or the *"Younger Than Springtime" Bufflehead*, is one of the most frequently encountered species of the *Denturus Calamitous Americanus* family. This feather-brained creature is generally a female who achieves full maturity during, or shortly after her menopause. Flush with insurance money gained from a recently buried husband, or full of the freedom and lust for further adventure that a substantial divorce settlement affords, this bird descends upon the prosthodontist full of heady visions of herself with new dentures.

The *Minewere Mallard* may be identified by her habit of flying backward—so that she can always see where she has been. Her mode of dress may be described as "teen twentyish" or more accurately, "nineteen twentyish." Positive identification is achieved when this beauty emits the shrill raucous call characteristic of the species. This is the *"Minewere"* or *"I Utsa"* sound, as in "Minewere always very white and small and perfect," or "I Usta look fuller in the face than this," or "Mine Usta fit tighter, Doctor!"

This creature harbors an image of herself which never existed, and can never be restored. Completely oblivious to the reality of her physical limitations, she naturally becomes disenchanted with her dentist. Her high hopes of regaining many lost years are unrealized and she seeks remedies of her own. It is not uncommon for these birds to place cotton under their lower dentures, or to line their cheeks with multiple sticks of chewing gum. The results are often grotesque and harmful. The "do-it-yourself" liners are the final step for these poor creatures, who have run out of dentists who will treat them. They spend their remaining days trying new nostrums, and busily changing the liners and plumpers on their dentures, as their ridges slowly shrink away.

Eternally Yours

Not all species of the *Denturus Calamitous Americanus* exhibit aggressive behavior. The *Forever Flicker* is a gentle creature with a chisel-shaped beak (for breaking through locked doors) and a heart full of love. This hardy cousin of the woodpecker, also known as the *Sweet-Lipped Sapsucker,* has an affinity for the dentist who has chronic duodenal ulcers and a short temper. Some instinct sends this bird in search of a dentist with a passion for order; the kind of man who likes to plan his treatment carefully, make the dentures, and complete a case. Once the right man has been spotted, this delicate creature nests in for a long stay. Generally she moves within walking distance of the office to save bus fare, but it is not uncommon for this species to make regular visitations over the years from quite a distance. This is the *Pilgrimage Variant* of the species.

Identification of the *Forever Flicker* can be made early if the dentist can hear this bird sing. If she is left alone in the chair for a while, one may hear a continuous, clear, double-noted warble that sounds unmistakably like "Till the End of Time." Without this clue, it is only possible to identify the bird after it is too late to matter.

This species is strictly a low pressure operator. There are no heartrending exclamations, no threats of legal action, and no comparisons with previous dentures. Ill will has no place in this lifetime liaison. Instead, there is an endless series of gentle complaints (say one per week) forever. The dentures always need adjusting, cleaning, sharpening, repairing, refitting, relieving, lightening, or tightening.

Specific instructions not to return, or extra charges for additional services are accepted with sweet tolerance and a patient smile by this persevering bird, because she knows something the dentist does not: only death will sever their relationship. It is simply a matter of who goes first.

The Gummy Rummies

The next group of difficult Denture Birds is an of-ten-encountered species. Because they vary so much in behavior and appearance, they are known by many names. Some of the more familiar are the *Tipsy Pipit*, the *Hollow-Legged Tanager*, the *Rummy Robin*, and the *Martini Meadowlark*. These feathered characters, together with their cousins (the *Heroin*, *Marijuana*, or *LSD Juncos*) form a colorful group whose numbers appear to be growing.

These playboys and girls display a wide variety of bizarre songs and markings. A common identi-fying characteristic, noted in all but the *Juncos*, is an affinity for spiritous liquids to the exclusion of other forms of nourishment. The odor of alcohol ac-companies every exhalation, and makes identifica-tion easy. Occasionally, these birds will reek of cologne or Bay Rum. One does not need to look hard for these free spirits, because they are found everywhere. They fly about on unsteady wings in search of a dentist who will make dentures which can float on their booze-ridden, fragile, and under-nourished oral tissues.

Unfortunately, these pathetic creatures cannot tolerate dentures without the constant support of their dentist, so that, unwittingly, he also becomes a part of their pattern of addiction.

The Woods Are Full of Them

These descriptions of a few species of the *Denturus Calamitous Americanus* are intended to sharpen the eyes of difficult denture bird watchers everywhere. There are many varieties yet to be described. The *Gagging Grackle* or the *Bruxing Booby* are often sighted. The *Ridge-less Firemouth Raven* is not an uncommon sight, and the *Whittling Denture Dove* has always been with us.

The woods are full of these unfortunate suffering individuals. They confound, frustrate, and antago-nize us, but their needs are so varied, and their problems so intense, that they stimulate and chal-lenge us to seek new ways to help them.

References

1. Schultz, A. W.: Management of Difficult Denture Patients. J Pros Dent 11:420, 1961.

2. Koper, A.: Why Dentures Fail. Dent Clin North Am 721–734, 1964.

3. Brewer, A. A.: Treating Complete Denture Patients. J Pros Dent 14:1015–1030, 1954.

DIFFICULT DENTURE BIRDS— NEW SIGHTINGS*

Alex Koper, D.D.S.

Difficult Denture Birds were first described in 1967.[1] These problem denture patients are individuals who complain, have pain, are hostile, tense, anxious, and unhappy people. They often exhibit regressive behavior and transfer many of their fears and frustrations to the mouth and face and endow their dentist with all sorts of unrealistic fantasies: he is an angel, a devil, a magician; he can be kind or cruel. The Difficult Denture Bird has been defined as a problem denture patient with much experience as a recipient of various kinds of dental therapy. He has developed a particularly colorful modus operandi that successfully thwarts efforts to provide dentures for him.

Wary Denture Bird watchers have reported new sightings of these colorful creatures over the years. They include the following species, readily recognized with hindsight.

Doctor, You're Good, But I Can Make Them Better

The *Whittling Denture Dove* and his cousin, *The Denture Sweller*, are experts in the art of diminishing and expanding the complete denture.

These are passive songsters who fill the dentist with nothing but praise until the dentures are complete. Amateur Denture Bird watchers occasionally confuse this species with the *Myway Magpie*[1] because both bird groups are preoccupied with the structural aspects of their dentures. The experienced observers who have encountered these lovelies know that the *Myway Magpies* busy themselves with the dentures only during the construction phase while the *Whittling Denture Dove* can hardly wait to get the finished dentures home to the workbench. Now the saws, files, and knives are whipped out and the dentures are "smoothed" and "evened up." At the slightest discomfort, out come the emery boards and away goes the denture base.

The *Denture Swellers* collect self-curing acrylic resin from drugstores like a nest-building bird collects straw and twigs. After gathering their brushes, files, and knives together, they take a fast look at themselves in the mirror and begin their plumping and facial contouring. The results of this creativity are often amazing and always destructive. Pleadings to let the dentist make the adjustments only stimulate further creative responses from these dental sculptors. They rarely return to their dentist until nothing remains to work with.

Grindings and Curses

The *Bruxing Booby* is a career bird. From his earliest days he has prepared himself for the role he will play when he finally has dentures to chew on. After wearing down his primary dentition and gnashing his permanent teeth away, he brings a lifetime of experience and overdeveloped masseter and pterygoid muscles to the encounter with dentures. The mutilation resulting to his overloaded and abused denture-bearing tissues brings howls of pain and threats of violence to the dentist. Day and night the grinding and cursing continue. As his residual alveolar ridges disintegrate and his bite (vertical dimension of occlusion) closes, more problems result.

One of the most unusual encounters this writer has had with a *Bruxing Booby* involved a chef who managed a busy kitchen in a large restaurant. He came in during his convalescence from gastric ulcer surgery, relaxed, calm, and reasonable. The warning signs of chronic ulcers, alcoholic breath, and a wife and children who could no longer live with him were overshadowed by his pleasant demeanor.

*Reprinted from the *Journal of Prosthetic Dentistry*, 60(1):70–74, 1988; with permission of Mosby, Inc.

His vertical dimension of occlusion was over-closed, his dentures were terribly underextended, and they had no retention. I was certain my dentures would succeed. They were completed, and he returned to work.

The problem was that when he worked he ground his teeth, fearfully and continuously, never stopping during this 2 PM-to-midnight period of busy, pressure-filled activity. He also sipped whiskey continuously, which not only calmed him but anesthetized him as well. The next morning he would awake with burning, traumatized tissues, run to this dentist full of pain and curses, and demand relief. After 34 adjustments and revisions, which included closing the occlusal vertical dimension of occlusion, my dentures looked just like his previous dentures. When I told him I could do no more for him he was outraged.

Bruxing Boobies never remove their dentures. They must grind and complain.

Heave Ho!

The *Gagging Grackle* dares the dentist to make dentures that he (the patient) cannot get rid of himself. The novice *Gagging Grackle* will upchuck during the impression stage and alert the dentist, thereby ending the game too soon. The novice also uses his hands occasionally to remove the dentures.

The experienced gagger learns that it is more fun to see how far one can toss the dentures when they are complete, so that the dentist does not find out about this patient's avocation until the day after the dentures are placed. Then the *Gagging Grackle* comes in with eyes filled with hate and brimming with tears. He tells about the work he is missing, the food he cannot eat, and his social embarrassment. It is all the dentist's fault, of course. The fact that he has never been able to wear dentures more than 15 minutes at a time is finally revealed and the usual disillusionment results. The dentist, filled with guilt, often refunds the patient his money, thus allowing him more adventures with other unwitting therapists.

I have found that the really expert denture chuckers compare favorably with other athletes such as discus or javelin throwers. Who knows, there may even be a denture-heaving competition in the Olympic Games of the future.

Doctor, I Have a Problem—Only You Can Help Me

A species of predator that has always been with us, whose presence is tacitly acknowledged but rarely discussed, is the *Family Paradisidae* or *Birds of Paradise.*

Credit for this sighting goes to Dr. Wayne Harvey (Personal communication, Denver, Colo., 1968), who described these creatures so well that I quote from his letter:

> "In the interest of bird watchers everywhere I should like to identify the *Family Paradisidae* or *Birds of Paradise*—a large species of very beautiful oscine birds. The members of this species are all female who are completely satisfied with their dentures. They have *other* problems which only the doctor can satisfy. I have heard that they are carnivorous.
>
> In our part of the world we call her a *Pink Breasted Bedthrasher.* You may recognize her by her distinctive, ear catching cry, 'coo-coo.'
>
> Be sure to keep your assistant with you at all times— particularly when she coos."

I am grateful to Dr. Harvey for this sighting. This bird is not an uncommon species and like the *Pink Breasted Bedthrasher,* is known by a variety of descriptive appellations such as the *Warm Bottomed Warbler* or the *Rigid Nippled Swift.*

One may see them flying about from office to office in their miniskirts, bosoms and thighs heaving, with a small mattress strapped to their backs. They carry a purse filled with erotic perfumes and seductive potions with slogans like "Instant Sex" painted on the outside in psychedelic colors. In his letter, Dr. Harvey mentioned that these birds are all female. This is because the males of this species die of exhaustion shortly after they reach puberty.

We all recognize the occupational hazards involved in treating these birds.

Paying Is Painful

The *Nopay Jay* is an expert at the art of getting something for as little as possible. His way of life is based on the premise that anyone can pay the fee for his dentures and conclude his professional relationship happily. The real skill involves getting the dentures and not paying for them.

There are a number of techniques used by these clever songsters. Most often they will delay payment of all but a token retainer. Occasionally they may drop a word or two about how well their oil wells are doing or the trouble they are having getting delivery on the new Rolls Royce they ordered some time ago. The dentist is complimented on his prowess, his consumate skill, his gentleness and understanding. Requests for payment are always accepted and deferred for one reason or another. Everyone has heard them: "I left my check book home." "The check is in the mail." "My husband is out of town and will send the money when he returns." The ploys are endless, delivered with the sincerity and skill that only experience can teach.

As soon as the dentures are placed, the trouble begins. Nothing is right, absolutely everything turned out different than it looked or felt at the final try-in. It hurts all over and besides it looks bad and this poor creature cannot talk. Time goes by, adjustment follows adjustment. Finally the *Nopay Jay* stops coming in altogether because the complication of a new malady, directly related to the dentures, makes a recluse of him. This illness, called "Autographic Paralysis," completely immobilizes the patient everytime he tries to write a check.

Notices and warnings of past due accounts are ignored, but when the pressure gets heavy enough, the patient strides into the office full of indignation, howling all kinds of new complaints and vowing never to pay until they are taken care of. The *Nopay Jay's* attorney threatens countersuit at the same time.

My last encounter with a *Nopay Jay* was 3 years ago with a lovely, wealthy widow 82 years of age. For a while I thought of waiting until my attorney could file a claim on her estate, but she is in excellent health and will live to be at least 100 years of age.

Litigious Songsters

There is the *Sweet Sue Sparrow* or the *I'llseeyouincourt Gull*, the most prolific breeders in the Difficult Denture Bird family today. They are filling the calendars of our courts with litigation, or at least threats of litigation, knowing that the cost of defense, the aggravation involved, and the dentist's time away from his practice often leads to unjustified settlements.

The *I'llseeyouincourt Gull* is generally a mature individual with time for litigious activities. A recent encounter of mine was with a gentleman whose grandson had recently graduated from law school and had just passed the California Bar examination. These birds thrive on controversy and enjoy the specter of their dentist writhing in agony in the unfamiliar environment of a courtroom.

Nonverbal Communicators

The *Aphasic Terns* are patients who seem to have great trouble communicating with their dentist during the treatment phase of denture fabrication, but as soon as the dentures are completed they become voluble experts at explaining every detail of countless problems.

To Dr. Charles A. Dodge (Personal communication, 1970) of Pleasant Hill, Calif. goes credit for a very accurate sighting of this species. He writes as follows:

"I would like to report another species that you may not have encountered to date.

This bird was female, 55 years of age, and principally distinguished by the fact that she was Portuguese. Although she had lived for many years in this country, she had never learned to speak English and so came accompanied by her 8-year-old granddaughter to act as interpreter.

Working under these handicaps I did the best denture service I could but was never really satisfied with the esthetics. Finally, however, in desperation I delivered the dentures. The next day the patient returned and was suddenly able to speak English and tell me all her complaints. She said that her husband didn't like her looks and so he tried them in and they didn't look good in him either. Faced with this over-whelming and indisputable evidence against me I set about to make another denture, and thanks to her newly acquired knowledge of the language, succeeded in pleasing the patient. I can only assume that the new set looked good in her husband, too.

An English-speaking variety of this bird is one that somehow manages to carry all the way through the denture series including the try-in phase and, despite all attempts of communication, fails to respond until final delivery, at which time the ability to describe the denture faults seems unlimited. Perhaps this is due to the new unrestricted tongue room provided by an increased vertical dimension of occlusion, together with correct contouring of the denture bases."

Dr. Dodge's description of an *Aphasic Tern* species that changes from a quiet Portuguese-speaking biddy to a loud-mouthed English squawking hen could only come from one who has had this experience.

This episode is the first time I have encountered dentures that can change a person's language. In addition, the dentist's ability to fit both the husband and the wife with one set of dentures is remarkable! It confirms my knowledge of his talents. He is, at least, a genius.

There are *Aphasic Terns* who communicate in writing, sign language, and in completely foreign tongues more effectively than if they could speak English—only, of course, until after the dentures are placed.

Who Needs Dentures!

The *Pocket Wearing Wren* is a fine, happy, male songster who just wants to be left alone. He has only one set of dentures and never comes in for adjustments because he hardly wears them. This wren is often away from home. He may be a fisherman, a beer salesman, a night watchman whose wife works days, or a mobile home repairman. The occupation is important because it allows him to pocket his dentures most of the time. When his wife is present, he is threatened with extinction unless he wears his teeth.

These birds eat everything from steak to popcorn with no dentition. They have excellent edentulous ridges and only had dentures made because of their spouses' insistence. The problem is not with the *Pocket Wearing Wren* but with the wives who blame their husbands' reluctance to wear dentures on the dentist—naturally.

Summary

Dr. Wes Hales (Personal communication) of San Francisco sums up the problem of dealing with Denture Birds eloquently when he says:

"The humor is a long way off when you deal with these birds. Sometimes you help them and bask in a little glory, but most just aggravate and frustrate you. In any event we plod along through ignorance and price and get stuck with them. Perhaps, as time goes by, we don't get stuck quite so often, but they get us now and then.

I hope the good Lord has a special place for us after all this, and perhaps, will make patients who need dentures in heaven with only beautiful ridges, healthy mouths, and well-coordinated tongues. That's assuming of course that we'll be there, too."

Reference

1. Koper A: Difficult denture birds. J Prosthet Dent 17:532–9, 1967.

MRS. DIVOT

For Better or For Worse*

Lynn Johnston

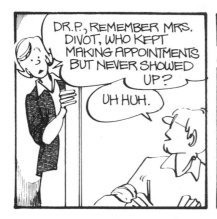

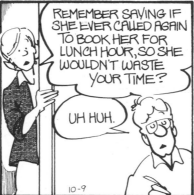

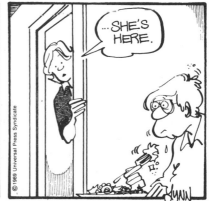

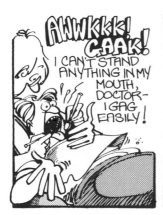

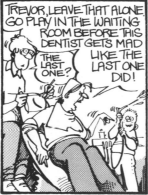

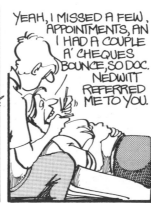

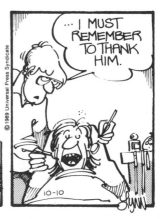

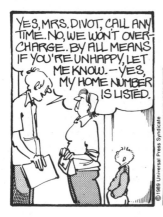

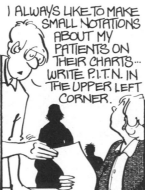

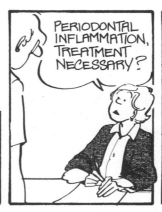

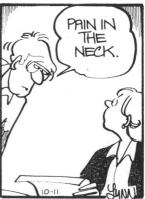

"HEY, DOC!"

Peter J. Schott

The school year—and my senior year—have begun. Apprehensions and uncertainties aside, I've decided to come fast off the mark in clinic this fall. You see, I have this burning desire to graduate.

Treating patients in a dental school setting is a tedious, obstacle-strewn ordeal that tries the most patient of souls. Often the slowness results not from the red tape and bureaucracy of the dental clinic, but from a lack of patient/doctor communication.

Behavioral science classes have beaten into us the need for good lines of communication in what they benignly call the "doctor/patient relationship." But they never told us about the language barrier. The problem is translating patientese into dentalese. I've spent hours trying to understand patients who are trying to understand dentistry.

Everybody has some good anecdotes on this subject. I could fill this entire issue with mine. I'd like to share just some of those priceless moments:

"Hey, Doc."
"Yes?"
"When are ya gonna gouge out my gums?"
"What?"
"You know, gouge them babies out."
"You mean the root planing and scaling?"
"No, Doc! The gum gouging! I think it's time for you to give my gums a real good bleed. I read about it in Reader's Digest."
"Are you sure it wasn't the *Enquirer*?"

"Doctor."
"Yes?"
"I changed my mind, I don't want this bridge after all."
"What! We're going to cement this next week!"
"No. I talked to my good friend Bob, and he said I should get a California bridge."
"Well, it's too late now and I think you mean a Maryland bridge. Besides, we talked about it and ruled it out in your treatment plan."
"Look, I know what I'm talking about. A California bridge! How do you think movie stars got sexy teeth? Bob had one made—no fuss, no muss. And he should know. He was stationed out in Hollywood when he was in the Navy."
"Great."
"I know you don't believe me. Do you want me to get Bob to come in and show you what I mean?"
"No, no, that's all right. I believe you and Bob."

"Excuse me, Doctor."
"What's up?"
"How come you never glued my son's teeth together?"
"Glued what?"
"Glued his teeth together. It's the latest thing. I hear you do that here."
"I'm not sure what you mean."
"I saw it on T.V. If you glue Johnny's back teeth together he won't get cavities."
"You mean pit and fissure sealants."
"No! Glue! Not fits and pressure. I'm tired of all the cavities he gets. He never brushes—stubborn like his father. While you're at it, glue his front teeth together so he won't get cavities there either."
"Whatever you want."

You can talk to them until you're blue in the face. You can explain treatment plans for hours on end. Some patients just can't get the drift of what's going on. Or else they blab incessantly about mysterious procedures they're sure you can perform.

In light of this, I want to write a patient/doctor dictionary to help those in our profession who aren't adept at translation. I'll have the latest jargon, gobbledygook, slang, and abbreviations for dental procedures all in one volume for easy refer-

*Reprinted with permission of the American Student Dental Association from *Dentistry85*, October 1985, pp 5–6.

ence. It will be published regionally to help dentists new to an area deal with strange pronunciations and expressions.

With a year to go and a lot of graduation requirements ahead of me, I wish I had one now. I'm so busy that I wonder if I'll ever have time to write my dental dictionary. Still, every day my hair goes gray trying to figure out what my patients want. And *I* want to graduate on time.

Forget the dictionary. I'm hiring a translator.

THE RELUCTANT PATIENT

Fox Trot*

Bill Amend

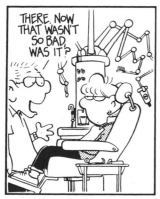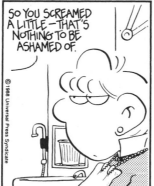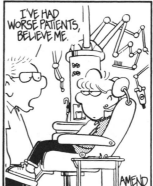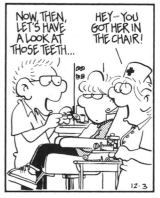

I AM JOE'S OVERHANG*

. . . A Fable

Paul R. Mahn, D.D.S.

I think it all began that Saturday morning at Dr. Cleene's suburban office. As slow as this day of the week always was, the doctor faithfully rendered himself available for a half-day for those who could not afford to take off work for their appointments. Oh yes—and for those children who could either not afford to take off from school, or could not afford to get hit in the face with a Saturday morning soccer ball. Anyway, I think that's when this whole thing started.

Dr. Cleene calmly entered the operatory. His young assistant, Beverly, had just seated his next patient. It was a very young patient. He knew this because no body parts projected from either side of the dental chair as he approached it from behind. Only the crisp, green corners of the paper napkin were visible slightly above the arms of the chair. A large woman, wearing an itchy brown topcoat, smothered the folding chair in the opposite corner of the room. Her Oil of Olay overcame the customary scent of formocresol.

"Ma'am, would you kindly step out into our reception area while we do Joey's filling?" Dr. Cleene asked. "I find it difficult to work if his attention is divided. Here . . . Bev will find you a magazine."

The woman scowled at the doctor as though he were her first morning cup of coffee. Bev promptly located an issue of *Fishing Facts.*

I was to be Joey's first silver filling. My wishes would have been to enter this world as an occlusal sealant—but no such luck. My destiny was predetermined by God . . . no, make that Insurance Coverage.

Dr. Cleene explained to the little boy (as he did to his mother over the phone) that he was going to make his tooth on the bottom fall asleep. He spoke to Joey in a quiet, friendly tone.

"When the tooth is asleep, Joey (carpule is loaded), I'll put a raincoat over your mouth (sy-

ringe is behind headrest), and I'll polish away the cavity so we can make a shiny filling (palpate the landmarks). Now . . . it'll prick just a little. . ."

The needle went in. Joey's limbs thrashed and his body bucked as he screamed and cursed in the guttural voice of a deceased ancestor. His head spun around 360° and his eyes fell deep into their sockets. Dr. Cleene was thrown back out of the operatory by some unseen force. He looked at the syringe. Only four-fifths of a carpule left. This kid must put a lot of sugar on his cereal. . .

Well, my account is getting a little long-winded here. Suffice it to say that, an hour later, "profound anesthesia was obtained"—okay? You fill in the details.

As Joey's energy apparently relented, it presented the doctor with a break to apply the rubber dam. Lubricant was not really necessary, for his lips were already covered with a uniform mucilage of grape Smucker's. Dr. Cleene tied on the clamp. Joey thrashed again, and the clamp ricocheted off of the overhead lamp—caromed off of Bev's forehead—and popped down Dr. Cleene's collar. Beverly leaned over and pulled on the long thread of floss coming out of Dr. Cleene's neckline, retrieving the projectile. Tiny red indentations on her forehead spelled out "IVORY."

After getting the dam in place, Dr. Cleene did the damn preparation. Joey's legs pumped like the pistons of an out-of-tune Chevy, and his screams behind the rubber dam resounded in a wet buzz.

It was three hours later when I was finally placed, condensed, and carved. I was not all that . . . handsome. Granted, it was hasty business—relative to the overall time frame. But I was more than an "MOD/A." I was a MONUMENT OF a DENTIST in the face of ADVERSITY. I can live with that, and I'm quite sure that Joey can.

Dr. Cleene complimented Joey on his champion

*Reprinted with permission from the *Wisconsin Dental Association Journal*, 63(12):694–697, 1987.

behavior, gave him a toy whistle, and adorned his t-shirt with a bright yellow sticker. It said "I AM A SUPER PATIENT." Dr. Cleene paved the way for the future.

That following month, Joey's family went vacationing at their cabin up north. On the second evening, Joey, in a total disregard for technology, cracked open a nutshell with his back teeth. His shiny "MOD" became an "MO" and a "DO." His family located a local dentist, and took him to visit the office the following morning.

Dr. Best stepped briskly into the operatory, looked at Joey's tooth (yes, Joey came in all by himself), and ordered a periapical radiograph. Joey meekly cooperated. After all, he'd had a dentist work on him once before, and it wasn't all that bad! The doctor then called Joey's mother and dad into the room.

"Joey's going to need a new filling. This one simply cannot be repaired."

I couldn't believe what I was hearing. I was marked for a one-way trip to the trap.

"Well, why did it break?" his dad asked. "I've bitten on nuts before, and I have a mouthful of fillings!"

"Well," Dr. Best replied, "the tooth was improperly prepared. And look at this radiogram—it's got a ragged overhang on each side. That's why his gums are so bleedy! Haven't you noticed that at all?"

Joey's mother began foaming at the mouth. "That filling was just done!"

Dr. Best replaced the filling while Joey's folks waited outside. They were confused. Why did Dr. Cleene leave those sharp edges hanging out? Why did he "prepare the tooth improperly" and still charge them the full amount? One-half hour later, Joey strutted out into the reception area with a new filling, and another sticker.

Once back home from their vacation, Joey's parents called Cleene's office. They demanded a full refund and an explanation, or they threatened to sue.

"And what was the problem with Dr. Cleene's work on Joey?" Beverly asked.

"The tooth was improperly prepared, of course!" came the father's reply. "Not to mention a 'hangover!' He ripped us off!"

Well, that's my account of the whole thing.

Joey's family got their money back and now see a different dentist (thanks to Dr. Best). Joey is now the model of fine behavior in the dental office (thanks to Dr. Cleene). And Dr. Cleene is seriously considering another line of work. Me? I'm buried in a scrap dump outside of New York City.

Is there an important lesson to be learned here? You bet there is:

"Sometimes you just have to be there."

And don't ever forget it. . .

THE VIEW FROM THE CHAIR:
Patients' Thoughts

Don't think for a minute that while patients are providing you with food for humor, you're not doing the same for them!

AN APPOINTMENT WITH THE DENTIST*

Gordon Harding

I just had my quarterly dental checkup. My second this century. My next one is set for the Year 2013. They gave me a slip of paper to remind me of the appointment.

The people in the dental office were astounded that I hadn't seen a dentist in 25 years. For my part, I was astounded that anyone willingly went more frequently. Who could have guessed that "quarterly" meant four times a *year?*

Actually the experience was kind of interesting. Doc found a popcorn hull we determined had been there since the bicentennial in '76. Then there was the caraway seed from 1969; the splinter from the stick of strawberry-flavored Good Humor purchased late in the summer of '67 in Chicago; and a variety of other things we couldn't identify or classify.

I'm older than Doc, so he was relying on me to label some of the things he dug out from between my teeth. Unfortunately, as one gets older, the memory is the first thing to go. That meant that some things remained a mystery.

I did remember when I had my last appointment. It was one of the few blanks on the medical/dental history form that I could fill out. That last visit to the dentist was either the summer of '62 or the fall of '63 in Webster City, Iowa. Or was it Fort Dodge? For that matter, was it Iowa?

I paused at the space labelled ALLERGIES and considered writing in "dentists," but I didn't think that attempt at levity would be well-received. In fact, laughing didn't seem to be in the forefront of anyone's mind. Doc said "Mmmmmmmm"a lot as he talked to his assistant in that special code peculiar to the dental trade. "Number 19—missing. Number 20, 21, 22—not worth mentioning. Number 23—" Well, you get the picture.

I don't want you to get the impression that I **fear** going to the dentist—but I think you must understand that some things take priority over dental checkups.

I didn't go in the late '60s because of the Vietnam War. Then there was the energy crisis in the '70s, plus Nixon, Watergate and the hostages in Iran. And frankly, with Reagan in the White House in the '80s, I didn't think there was any point in making commitments like dental appointments. And I moved around a lot

My life has slowed a little and I thought I should take advantage of this brief period of stability (I've lived in Randolph for the past 16 years) and get my teeth checked.

The modern dentist has got his act together. The last dentist I went to worked with implements made by Craftsman that had lifetime guarantees.

And there have been other changes.

I didn't know that dentists no longer give haircuts, for example.

But I think I appreciated the subtle changes the most. I hardly ever saw the dentist or his assistant. They sat behind me—out of sight, out of mind.

Twenty-five years ago, the dentist seemed to be crawling in my lap. He'd pull his toolbox right up in front of me, then swing the porcelain tray right under my nose and load that baby up with the meanest collection of twisted tools I ever saw. And hanging right over my head was that quadruple jointed monster with the funny belts that made a whining sound and produced smoke in my oral cavity. And pain. I remember the pain.

Doc never showed me the modern version, and I'm grateful for that act of kindness. Regardless of what it looked like, it sounded quite pleasant. Merely hummed. And no pain.

The chair itself has undergone significant change. The straps are missing, for example. And the new chairs don't really have proper armrests. Nothing you can get a good grip on. I used to leave permanent fingerprints on the chairs a quarter-century ago. I used to surprise dentists with my strength.

*Reprinted with permission from the *Vermont State Dental Society Newsletter*, (June): 1988.

They've even changed the toothbrushes. When I was a kid, a toothbrush had some permanence. If you were lucky, you would get a toothbrush for Christmas. The one I had was indestructible. I later used it for removing body rust on my 1939 Plymouth convertible coupe. It still gets pulled out of my toolbox whenever I'm cleaning copper fittings during spurts of recreational sweat soldering.

Last week, Doc gave me a brand new toothbrush with soft bristles and told me I've been brushing my teeth wrong for all these years. That, I guess, explains a lot.

I wonder where I put that appointment slip?

A CHILD'S-EYE VIEW OF DENTISTRY*

What do children really think about the dentist? A group of seven- and eight-year-olds at the Smith-Barnes Elementary School in Stockbridge, GA, were asked to do drawings. One by Jason Armistead appears here.—Ed.

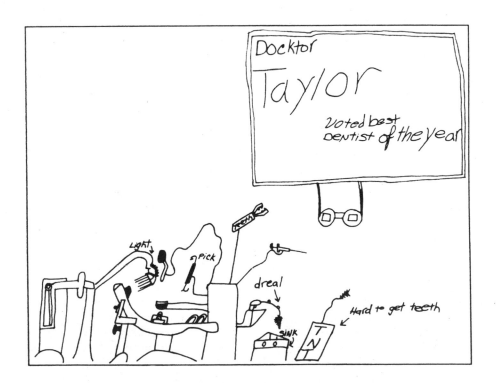

*Reprinted with permission from the American Student Dental Association, Chicago; from *Dentistry87*, December 1987.

TRADING PLACES*

When the Doctor Goes to the Dentist

Perri Klass, M.D.

I just want to make it clear that when I asked the dentist whether I could have my wisdom teeth out in the morning and then go on to work, I wasn't trying to be funny.

You have to understand, I've always enjoyed fairly rude good health. I see a doctor only when I'm pregnant; I never have my cholesterol checked. As a pediatrician, I'm concerned with things that can go wrong with children's bodies, not my own. And because I never have cavities, I don't think about the dentist very much at all. Now I could lie and say I never have cavities because I brush properly and floss daily and avoid refined sugars. But the truth is, I seem to have good genes where teeth are concerned—and that counts for a lot. Nevertheless, in my unflossed, candy-eating good fortune, I do at times feel mildly self-righteous about not getting cavities, as though the strength of my teeth must reflect some shining virtue in my soul.

So I go to the dentist every six months or so to have my teeth cleaned, to be told I have no cavities and to be reminded to floss regularly. I'm a big baby about having my teeth cleaned—my lack of experience with fillings has left me very wary of anyone coming near my mouth with instruments. Sometime during my medical residency I discovered the joys of nitrous oxide, and ever since, I've had my teeth cleaned while I was under laughing gas. As a resident I would go to sleep as soon as they put the gas mask on my face; of course, in those days I existed in a state of constant fatigue, and just reclining in a cushioned chair would send me off at any hour of the day or night.

Anyway, this dentist I went to recently had convinced me it was time to have two of my wisdom teeth out, and I was happy to hear he was going to give me nitrous oxide when he pulled them. When I asked him whether I would be able to go on to work afterward, he looked a little dubious. "Well,"

he said, "wait and see how you feel." I figured I would have my teeth out at ten, finish by eleven and get to work by early afternoon.

Clearly, I had no idea what's involved in having wisdom teeth out. I didn't know whether it was a big deal, a small deal or a medium-sized deal, so I assumed it was a very small deal indeed.

I lay back in the chair. After giving me a short lecture about how I would feel no pain, only pressure, he put the mask over my face. He injected me with Novocain. And then there was this truly incredible pressure—pressure so beyond anything the word suggests that I can only consider it a kind of pain. Even though one part of my brain was outraged by the sensations I was being subjected to, thanks to the nitrous oxide I was mostly just mildly amused by the whole thing.

After I spent a spell in Nitrous Land, the dentist triumphantly showed me the first tooth: one down, one to go. I made a comment that seemed to me rather witty, but it was unfortunately—or perhaps fortunately—muffled by the gas mask, and therefore lost to posterity.

The second tooth, nitrous or no nitrous, seemed to be taking a lot longer than the first. I opened my eyes and noticed the dentist's forehead was covered with beads of sweat. He explained some problem, and I listened but from a misty distance. If you're someone like me who does not habitually use any mind-altering substance more powerful than a glass of wine, nitrous oxide qualifies as a major hallucinogen. So I smiled and nodded when he said he'd have to pull this tooth out in pieces. What with one thing and another, it took more than an hour.

When he was done and I sat up, the first inkling I had that I'd been through something more than the usual was after I asked whether he ever used general anesthesia for extractions. He told me yes, he did for very bad ones, and he guessed mine had

*Reprinted from *American Health,* (May): 96, 99, 1992.

been in that category—maybe I should have had general anesthesia. "Don't be silly," I said, as he packed my mouth with gauze. "I'm just fine." And I made some self-congratulatory remark about how, after childbirth, this was nothing. The dentist gave me a prescription for painkillers, which I tucked into my pocket.

And then I drove to work, bloody gauze and all. Why not? But with my head throbbing and my battered jaw feeling as though it was about to come loose, I began to think about why not. When I got to work, I changed the gauze pads for fresh ones and began to tell my story to my colleagues.

My jaw hurt an awful lot for the next few days. Naturally—despite my extensive preparation in pathophysiology and anatomy—I had not expected that pain, had not planned for it. I had things to do and places to go and hard, crusty things to eat. But here I was, totally dependent on pain pills, carefully calculating when I could take the ones that really worked but affected my judgment and my driving, and when I would have to get by on ibuprofen, which left me with a clear brain but an aching jaw.

The truth is, on some level I don't believe in painkillers. I tell myself that if I keep busy, concentrate on other things, the pain will go away. It's part and parcel of not attending to my own medical needs, I suppose. We doctors deny in ourselves the "frailties" we spend our lives confronting in others.

To add insult to injury, my jaw did not heal properly. I developed something called dry-socket syndrome and had to wait about a week before tissue grew over the exposed extraction site to cover and protect it.

Being in pretty bad pain chronically for days didn't do good things for my disposition. I was grouchy, snappish and full of self-pity—and above all, I felt entitled. I mean, whatever I was doing at any particular moment, wasn't I a saint to be doing it? Packing my kids' lunches—what a mom! Never a thought for herself as her head throbs with the agonies of hell. Asking another mother about her baby's diarrhea—wasn't I a selfless physician! And

so on, until things calmed down and I could take another pain pill.

I am not at all pleased to dwell upon the thought that almost every doctor is some other doctor's patient. Doctors are, in fact, bad patients, notoriously negligent about following their own advice. In a recent survey of physicians on the Harvard Medical School faculty, doctors got good grades for wearing seat belts and abstaining from smoking. They were much weaker, however, on the diet and exercise front, and they seemed to be as frightened of needles as their patients were. Many were not even immunized against hepatitis B and influenza, diseases they risk exposure to in the course of practicing medicine.

Generally, we doctors fall into two categories of behavior as patients: hysterical hypochondria and relentless denial. The hypochondriac is particularly common in medical school, where students, totally immersed in a medical environment, discover they have all the classic symptoms of one disease after another. Occasional diarrhea becomes inflammatory bowel disease. The lingering headache is symptomatic of a brain tumor. Exhaustion may well be chronic fatigue syndrome or the early stages of African sleeping sickness.

But as we move on from training to real life as doctors, the trend often shifts toward denial. I believed that if I ignored the pain in my tooth rather than coddling it with analgesics, it would go away. I should have known better. Medicine is full of stories about doctors who ignore pain in their chests, lumps in their breasts and other intimations of possible serious illness. Knowing what a symptom might mean does not necessarily guarantee you'll respond to it rationally and promptly—not even when you're a doctor.

Not so long ago—having recovered from my dental woes—I managed to miss the first doctor appointment I had made in years. Something came up at work. Something about a patient. You know, a patient—a *sick* person. A person who needs a doctor—not someone like me.

NOW OPEN EVEN WIDER . . .

The Far Side*

Gary Larson

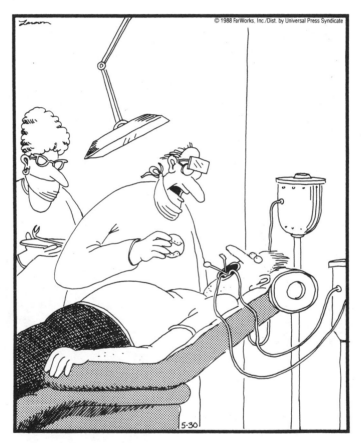

"Now open even wider, Mr. Stevens. . . . Just out of curiosity, we're going to see if we can also cram in this tennis ball.

ENCLOSED WITH A CHECK FROM A PATIENT*

Roger Duncan

To My Dentist:

When I smile at Mrs. Jones, I think of you.
When I eat my Grapenut stones, I think of you.
When I see my children's grins
And my lovey's dental pins,
When I recall our loud guffaws
At your sterile belligerent paws,
And the bright belligerent faces
Of your staff in all their places,
I smile, and my day though hard and crappy
Seems better—and a bit more happy.
I feel a tad bit ill
Because I can't pay ALL my bill,
But I someday will.

*Reprinted with permission from the *Journal of the Colorado Dental Association*, (Autumn): 34, 1991.

NOTHING BUT THE TOOTH*

S. J. Perelman

I am thirty-eight years old, have curly brown hair and blue eyes, own a uke and a yellow roadster, and am considered a snappy dresser in my crowd. But the thing I want most in the world for my birthday is a free subscription to *Oral Hygiene*, published by Merwin B. Massol, 1005 Liberty Avenue, Pittsburgh, Pa. In the event you have been repairing your own teeth, *Oral Hygiene* is a respectable smooth-finish technical magazine circulated to your dentist with the compliments of his local supply company. Through its pages runs a recital of the most horrendous and fantastic deviations from the dental norm. It is a confessional in which dentists take down their back hair and stammer out the secrets of their craft. But every time I plunge into its crackling pages at my dentist's, just as I get interested in the story of the Man with the Alveolar Dentures or Thirty Reasons Why People Stay Away from Dentists, the nurse comes out slightly flushed and smoothing her hair to tell me that the doctor is ready. Last Thursday, for example, I was head over heels in the question-and-answer department of *Oral Hygiene*. A frankly puzzled extractionist, who tried to cloak his agitation under the initials "J.S.G.," had put his plight squarely up to the editor: "I have a patient, a woman of 20, who has a full complement of teeth. All of her restorations are gold foils or inlays. She constantly grinds her teeth at night. How can I aid her to stop grinding them? Would it do any good to give her a vellum rubber bite?" But before I could learn whether it was a bite or just a gentle hug the editor recommended, out popped Miss Inchbald with lipstick on her nose, giggling, "The Doctor is free now." Free, indeed—"running amok" would be a better way to put it.

I had always thought of dentists as of the phlegmatic type—square-jawed sadists in white aprons who found release in trying out new kinds of burs on my shaky little incisors. One look at *Oral Hygiene* fixed that. Of all the inhibited, timorous, uncertain fumble-bunnies who creep the earth, Mr. Average Dentist is the worst. A filing clerk is a veritable saber-toothed tiger by comparison. Faced with a decision, your dentist's bones turn to water and he becomes all hands and feet. He muddles through his ordinary routine with a certain amount of bravado, plugging a molar here with chewing gum, sinking a shaft in a sound tooth there. In his spare time he putters around his laboratory making tiny cement cupcakes, substituting amber electric bulbs for ordinary bulbs in his waiting room to depress patients, and jotting down nasty little innuendoes about people's gums in his notebook. But let an honest-to-goodness sufferer stagger in with his face out of drawing, and Mr. Average Dentist's nerves go to hell. He runs sobbing to the "Ask *Oral Hygiene*" department and buries his head in the lap of V. C. Smedley, its director. I dip in for a typical sample:

Question—A patient of mine, a girl, 18, returned from school recently with a weird story of lightning having struck an upper right cuspid tooth and checked the enamel on the labial surface nearly two-thirds of the way from the incisal edge toward the neck. The patient was lying on a bed looking out an open window during an electric storm, and this one flash put out the lights of the house, and at the same time, the patient felt a burning sensation (like a burning wire) along the cuspid tooth. She immediately put her tongue on the tooth which felt rough, but as the lights were out she could not see it so she went to bed. (A taste as from a burnt match accompanied the shock.)

Next morning she found the labial of the tooth black. Some of the color came off on her finger. By continually brushing all day with the aid of peroxide, salt, soda and vinegar she removed the remainder of the black after which the tooth was a yellow shade and there was some roughness on the labial surface.

Could the lightning have caused this and do you recommend smoothing the surface with discs?
—R. D. L., D.D.S., Oregon

Well, Doctor, let us take your story step by step. Miss Muffet told you the sensation was like a burning wire, and she tasted something like a burnt match. Did you think, by any chance, of looking into her mouth for either wire or matches? Did you even think of looking into her mouth? I see no mention of the fact in your letter. You state that she walked in and told you the story, that's all. Of course it never occurred to you that she had brought along her mouth for a reason. Then you say, "she removed the remainder of the black after which the tooth was a yellow shade." Would it be asking too much of you to make up your mind? Was it a tooth or a yellow shade? You're quite sure it wasn't a Venetian blind? Or a gaily striped awning? Do you ever take a drink in the daytime, Doctor?

Frankly, men, I have no patience with such idiotic professional behavior. An 18-year-old girl walks into a dentist's office exhibiting obvious symptoms of religious hysteria (stigmata, etc.). She babbles vaguely of thunderstorms and is patently a confirmed drunkard. The dentist goes to pieces, forgets to look in her mouth, and scurries off to *Oral Hygiene* asking for permission to smooth her surface with discs. It's a mercy he doesn't take matters into his own hands and try to plow every fourth tooth under. This is the kind of man to whom we entrust our daughters' dentures.

There is practically no problem so simple that it cannot confuse a dentist. For instance, thumb-sucking. "Could you suggest a method to correct thumb and index finger sucking by an infant of one year?" flutters a Minnesota orthodontist, awkwardly digging his toe into the hot sand. Dr. Smed-

ley, whose patience rivals Job's, has an answer for everything: "Enclose the hand by tying shut the end of the sleeve of a sleeping garment, or fasten a section of a pasteboard mailing tube to the sleeping garment in such a position as to prevent the bending of the elbow sufficiently to carry the thumb or index finger to the mouth." Now truly, Dr. Smedley, isn't that going all the way around Robin Hood's barn? Nailing the baby's hand to the highchair is much more cozy, or, if no nail is available, a smart blow with the hammer on Baby's fingers will slow him down. My grandfather, who was rather active in the nineties (between Columbus and Amsterdam avenues—they finally got him for breaking and entering), always used an effective method to break children of this habit. He used to tie a Mills grenade to the baby's thumb with cobbler's waxed thread, and when the little spanker pulled out the detonating pin with his teeth, Grandpa would stuff his fingers into his ears and run like the wind. Ironically enough, the people with whom Grandpa now boards have the same trouble keeping him from biting his thumbs, but overcome it by making him wear a loose jacket with very long sleeves, which they tie to the bars.

I have always been the mildest of men, but you remember the old saying, "Beware the fury of a patient man." (I remembered it very well and put my finger on it instantly, page 269 of Bartlett's book of quotations.) For years I have let dentists ride roughshod over my teeth; I have been sawed, hacked, chopped, whittled, bewitched, bewildered, tattooed, and signed on again; but this is cuspid's last stand. They'll never get me into that chair again. I'll dispose of my teeth as I see fit, and after they're gone, I'll get along. I started off living on gruel, and, by God, I can always go back to it again.

THIS IS GOING TO HURT JUST A LITTLE BIT*

Ogden Nash

One thing I like less than most things is sitting in a
dentist chair with my mouth wide open,
And that I will never have to do it again is a hope
that I am against hope hopen.
Because some tortures are physical and some are
mental,
But the one that is both is dental.
It is hard to be self-possessed
With your jaw digging into your chest,
So hard to retain your calm
When your fingernails are making serious
alterations in your life line or love line or some
other important line in your palm;
So hard to give your usual effect of cheery
benignity
When you know your position is one of the two or
three in life lacking in dignity.
And your mouth is like a section of road that is
being worked on.
And it is all cluttered up with stone crushers and
concrete mixers drills and steam rollers and
there isn't a nerve in your head that you aren't
being irked on.
Oh, some people are unfortunate enough to be
strung up by thumbs,
And others have things done to their gums,
And your teeth are supposed to be being polished,
But you have reason to believe they are being
demolished,

And the circumstance that adds most to your
terror
Is that it's all done with a mirror,
Because the dentist may be a bear, or as the
Romans used to say, only they were referring to
a feminine bear when they said it, an *ursa*,
But all the same how can you be sure when he
takes his crowbar in one hand and mirror in the
other he won't get mixed up, the way you do
when you try to tie a bow tie with the aid of a
mirror, and forget that left is right and *vice
versa?*
And then at last he says That will be all; but it isn't
because he then coats your mouth from cellar to
roof
With something that I suspect is generally used to
put a shine on a horse's hoof.
And you totter to your feet and think, Well it's all
over now and after all it was only this once,
And he says come back in three monce.
And this, O Fate, is I think the most vicious circle
that thou ever sentest,
That Man has to go continually to the dentist to
keep his teeth in good condition when the chief
reason he wants his teeth in good condition is
so that he won't have to go to the dentist.

*Reprinted from *The Face is Familiar* by Ogden Nash; © 1938 by
Ogden Nash; with permission of Little, Brown, and Company.

The two following papers originally appeared separately in the Chico News and Review. *Dr. Campbell's writing was published in response to Mr. Stout's article.—Ed*

TYRANTS OF TEETH*

Robert Joe Stout

I don't drink much hard liquor, and never have a bottle of it around. But that night 2 months ago, I wished that I did—I'd've slugged down anything to mute the pain. I'd already taken aspirin, but the throbbing was so severe I couldn't come close to sleep.

Had it been daylight I might even have gone to a dentist.

Finally, I dozed off. And though the tooth bothered me the next day, the pain never got so severe that I had to pick up the telephone and make an appointment. I don't know which dentist I would have called anyway. They're all the same.

Dentists, like veterinarians, have emerged from being public servants to becoming public tyrants. Whatever humility they might have grown up with they leave in dental school. Twenty-five years ago, when one had a problem with a tooth, one got it pulled or filled. Now one gets a lecture, a lesson on brushing, a set of x-rays, a lot of questions about one's personal finances and insurance and a reference slip to another dentist who specializes in gum care or root canals or reconstructive bridges.

Not, mind you, that they're not professionally adept. Technically they can do things that dentists 25 years ago couldn't do. They can save teeth, rebuild teeth, straighten teeth, rearrange teeth, but in the process of attaining those new abilities they seem to have lost a very important old one: the ability to understand that some of us—many of us—don't care whether or not we look like Burt Reynolds, or have a perfect bite, or keep our mouths filled with reinforced enamel.

We simply want to be able to eat—and sleep—without pain.

We want to say, "Look, I've got $40. Do what you can for the cash."

Unfortunately, it's hard as hell to find a dentist who'll do that. Dentists today regard each mouth as an aesthetic challenge. They're not, they'll explain, mere mechanics—on, no! They react with shocked horror if you even, politely, suggest that they do a bit of emergency work. They jump up on their soapbox and expound the philosophy of the new dentistry. They make it quite plain that you, poor plebian, have no rights, no intelligence, no sensibilities. They shame you into $3,000 worth of dental work you can't afford.

"What?" they'll feign surprise. "No insurance? Did you bring the deed to your house?"

I suppose though, despite my dislikes, they're doing me a favor. I've nursed the tooth for months by not eating sweets. I've chewed my food conscientiously, avoided beverages that are either too hot or too cold and carefully brushed and flossed for anything that might put pressure on the aching bastard.

But I still resent feeling that I can't get the repairs that I want done. I want to be master of my own mouth. I want to decide whether I spend the scarce dollars I earn on a dentist's Porsche or my daughter's typewriter. I want an open market, not carbon copies who endlessly repeat the same cliches.

I want to go to sleep tonight knowing that I can afford breakfast in the morning.

*Reprinted with permission of *Chico News and Review.

TYRANTS OF TYPE*

Kevin Campbell, D.D.S.

I'm just your average dentist. I watch a little TV. I don't read trashy novels. I do read the newspapers, but I stay away from the editorial page, from movie and restaurant reviews; even, sad to say, theatre and book reviews lately. I'm finding them increasingly inaccurate, canted usually to the negative. Often, the honest effort of others is dispensed with too easily in a neat 500-word essay, just for the sake of a good story. It makes me uncomfortable. It's usually done so glibly.

Imagine my chagrin then, when I perused my appointment book the other morning and found that a columnist (!) was coming to my office. Myra, the receptionist, must have been daydreaming when she made that appointment. A telephone number was written below his name. I was tempted to call and find out what paper he "wrote" for, but I knew I'd be wasting my time. Columnists are all the same.

In fact, columnists, like interior decorators, have emerged from being public servants to becoming public tyrants. Whatever sensibility or sensitivity they might have grown up with they left in undergrad English and journalism classes long ago. Instead of studying, they drank themselves into an alcoholic stupor night after night, until their livers were mush, and the intricate protein pathways of their brains sclerosed into superhighways of cynicism. Tragically, because of these habits, they could not go on to graduate school. They had to settle for being columnists. Their mission in life? To give us all a headache whether we've been drinking or not.

I'm not saying that columnists aren't professionally adept. They can turn a phrase as well as the next technical manual writer. Indeed, they can whip out a 500-word essay faster than a freshman at finals time, and usually make just as much sense.

Some columnists even do their research. Unfortunately, it's hard to find one of these. It's not only alcohol. It's TV. Poor souls, they have to compete with those brisk, flashy special reports and personality commentaries. When they try to do this they feel guilty, then resentful, and as you have seen, the resentment shows. It's not the urge to cop out. It's the failure to cop out. They don't even own a suit good enough to wear on TV! Also, most of them suffer from columnist's nose, a disease too painful to discuss here.

We tried to cancel the appointment but his column wasn't due until the next day so he'd stayed at home watching "Leave It to Beaver" reruns. His phone was disconnected. He simply couldn't be reached.

I became very anxious. Despite the fact that I'd spent 8 years earning my degree, including the humiliation of my freshman year in dental school; despite the fact that I complete 50 units of continuing education every 2 years to stay current with my profession; yes, despite the fact that my profession ranks below only the clergy in public respect and trust (a fact that could only be learned through research), my career was about to be ruined.

A columnist was coming to visit. A columnist in pain! I'd rather have confronted a raging bull elephant.

I panicked! I had to do something to drive him off. I called my friend, Joe the plumber, and convinced him to park his Porsche in my spot. I made the columnist sign a lien against his house, subordinating Bank of America, to insure payment for treatment. I asked my mother-in-law to impersonate the hygienist, and then told her the columnist was my best drinking pal. But nothing stopped him.

In the end, despite my best efforts, I had to see him. My worst fears were confirmed. He had an abscessed tooth. I had to tell him I could save it. I was ethically compelled. Since he asked, I also had to tell him what it would cost, in terms of time and money. I would rather serve tea to a Tory. He screamed at me. "I bet you send people to specialists! I bet you try to save their teeth just because

*Reprinted with permission of *Chico News and Review*.

modern research has given you the tools to do so! Just so you can say you tried your best! I'm on to your tricks! I'm gonna spend my money on a color TV!"

Well, it was a painful week. I had to read his column every day. I was compelled to watch him mix his hatred and suspicion of me with his own self-pity, his repressed hatred of his mother, his disappointment in his father, and his career frustrations in general.

But since that week, life has gone on as usual.

I've stopped reading the columnists again—the reviews, the editorials. I don't want to watch them mix their hatred and suspicion of ballplayers, and chefs (in fact, of anyone who figures they can do better than writing an occasional 500-word essay) with all their repressed hostility. The way I figure it, if reading them constitutes being informed, ignorance is bliss.

By the way, in case any of you columnists are out there reading this story, it's called a parody.

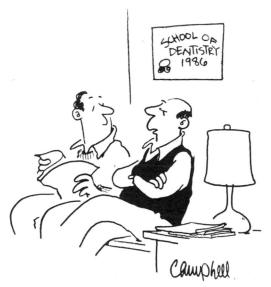

"I like young dentists. Their stories are shorter."

Martha Campbell*

LESSONS IN PRACTICE MANAGEMENT

Unlike physicians, the majority of dentists are not dependent on an institutional setting, such as a hospital, to provide care. Most of us work in solo practices. While we have almost total control of our practices (excluding regulatory agencies—see Dentistry, the Law, and Regulation), we sacrifice regular interactions with colleagues. Because of this isolation, we manage our practices in different ways. Amazingly, most of us learn the skills necessary to accomplish this by a combination of trial and error and advice from peers. Alternatively, some of us turn to the burgeoning industry of continuing education courses, where we learn how to earn a million dollars a week while seeing patients on alternate Tuesdays when there is a full moon. This section covers a variety of topics that should ring familiar.

THE TWELVE DAYS OF PRACTICE*

Martin T. Nweeia, D.D.S.

1

On the first day of practice
My country gave to me

Health reform
That no one can agree.

2

On the second day of practice
My country gave to me

Two HMO'S,
And health reform
That no one can agree.

3

On the third day of practice
My country gave to me

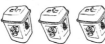

Three sharps containers,
Two HMO'S,
And health reform
That no one can agree.

4

On the fourth day of practice
My country gave to me

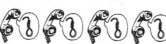

Four lawyers calling,
Three sharps containers,
Two HMO'S,
And health reform
That no one can agree.

5

On the fifth day of practice
My country gave to me

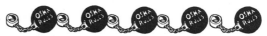

Five new OSHA rules,
Four lawyers calling,
Three sharps containers,
Two HMO'S,
And health reform
That no one can agree.

6

On the sixth day of practice
My country gave to me

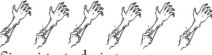

Six assistants gloving,
Five new OSHA rules,
Four lawyers calling,
Three sharps containers,
Two HMO'S,
And health reform
That no one can agree.

7

On the seventh day of practice
My country gave to me

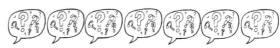

Seven questions,
"Is your equipment sterile, doctor?"
Six assistants gloving,
Five new OSHA rules,
Four lawyers calling,
Three sharps containers,
Two HMO'S,
And health reform
That no one can agree.

*Reprinted with permission of the *Hawaii Dental Journal,* (Dec): 6-7, 1993; graphics by Kevin Hand.

8

On the eighth day of practice
My country gave to me

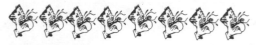

Eight patients gagging,
Seven questions,
  "Is your equipment sterile, doctor?"
Six assistants gloving,
Five new OSHA rules,
Four lawyers calling,
Three sharps containers,
Two HMO'S,
And health reform
That no one can agree.

9

On the ninth day of practice
My country gave to me

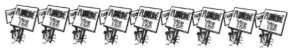

Nine fluoride activists,
Eight patients gagging,
Seven questions,
  "Is your equipment sterile, doctor?"
Six assistants gloving,
Five new OSHA rules,
Four lawyers calling,
Three sharps containers,
Two HMO'S,
And health reform
That no one can agree.

10

On the tenth day of practice
My country gave to me

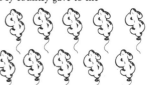

Ten overhead costs a'rising,
Nine fluoride activists,
Eight patients gagging,
Seven questions,
  "Is your equipment sterile, doctor?"
Six assistants gloving,
Five new OSHA rules,
Four lawyers calling,
Three sharps containers,
Two HMO'S,
And health reform
That no one can agree.

11

On the eleventh day of practice
My country gave to me

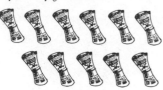

Eleven misleading media reports,
Ten overhead costs a'rising,
Nine fluoride activists,
Eight patients gagging,
Seven questions,
  "Is your equipment sterile, doctor?"
Six assistants gloving,
Five new OSHA rules,
Four lawyers calling,
Three sharps containers,
Two HMO'S,
And health reform
That no one can agree.

12

On he twelfth day of practice
My country gave to me

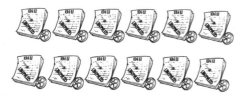

Twelve unapproved insurance claims
Eleven misleading media reports,
Ten overhead costs a'rising,
Nine fluoride activists,
Eight patients gagging,
Seven questions,
  "Is your equipment sterile, doctor?"
Six assistants gloving,
Five new OSHA rules,
Four lawyers calling,
Three sharps containers,
Two HMO'S,
And health reform
That no one can agree.

By the thirteenth day of practice
My profession struggles to be
The caring art that first attracted me.

10 TERRIFIC WAYS TO ANSWER THE CALLER WHO ASKS "HOW MUCH DO YOU CHARGE FOR A ROOT CANAL?"*

Richard S. Winters, D.D.S.

With increasing frequency we have been receiving calls asking about our fees for Root Canal Therapy. The consumer has become so cost-conscious in all areas that the medical and dental professions have become fair game for such questions.

First of all, I hate the question. A root canal is not a finite product that can be purchased like the proverbial "can of peas." My expertise may be better or worse than someone else's. Be assured, the callers are quite sophisticated from shopping around and know the difference between an anterior tooth and a molar. They also have become more brazen such as the fellow who belligerently asks my secretary "How much do you charge for a molar root canal?" If she replies with a dollar figure that he doesn't like, he slams the phone down. Or, if she states that the doctor would like to see him to evaluate the condition of the tooth, he answers "I called your competitors and they all gave me a price!"

Let us assume that the caller has a right to ask us to quote our fees, which he or she does. How do we answer this question intelligently? We will endeavor here to list different approaches which will try to reconcile our professional pride with the buyer's right to know.

1. Quote your usual and customary fee, assuming the caller knows a lateral from a third molar. If the caller replies, "WHAT! I can take a trip to Europe for that kind of money," tell him to book the flight immediately as the fares may soon go up.

2. Ask the caller what his lowest quoted fee was. The caller will abruptly hang up on you.

3. Tell the caller "We don't quote fees over the phone." He will abruptly hang up and call the Board of Dentistry to report you.

4. Quote the fee that your friend who practices on Central Park South in New York City tells you he charges. The caller will abruptly hang up.

5. Ask the caller what he considers a fair fee. If he tells you that his mother-in-law had a molar root canal for $65, tell him to go where his mother-in-law went. Hopefully, she is still alive or you may be sued for phone abuse.

6. Offer for free: An exam, a full series of X-rays, a cleaning, six tubes of Sensodyne and a ticket to a New Jersey Nets game—if only the patient will come in.

7. Ask the caller who referred him to your office. If he answers with the name of someone you know and like, tell him everything—come clean. However, if it's someone you never heard of or dislike, or if it is Lorena Bobbitt or the Menendez Brothers, tell him that you are solidly booked for a month and do not work on days ending in the letter "Y."

8. Tell the caller that your fees are competitive with those of other dentists in the area. He will tell you that he is going to report you for collusion and abruptly hang up.

9. If the caller says he found you in the Yellow Pages, tell him everything he wants to know about anything: your fees, where you bought your car, your sex life, anything. I wouldn't fool around when it comes to the Yellow Pages.

10. If a woman calls and tells you that she just moved here from Nebraska and she needs root canals on her anteriors, bicuspids and molars—beware! She works for a dentist and wants to know your fees so she can figure out what to tell callers

*Reprinted with permission from the *Journal of the New Jersey Dental Association*, (Winter):67–68, 1995.

who want to know "How much do you charge for root canal?"

Summary

Various ways of answering this question have been presented with responses to each. You can use any or all of the cited examples or make up some of your own.

Conclusion

After trying to figure out a way to answer this question intelligently, and trying to accommodate all callers, we have found that whatever we say the caller does not make an appointment. It has become a lesson in futility. I must assume that someone out there must be treating these people. Who is it? What do you say to them? Please let me know. All responses will be confidential.

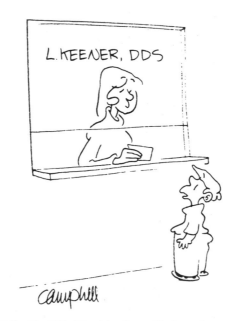

"Hello. I'm Billy Hendrix, the cyclical earnings peak."

Martha Campbell*

A DOSE OF THEIR OWN MEDICINE*

This is an exchange between Dr. Lawson Broadrick and a claims service examiner. Most of you are too familiar with the contents of the first letter. However, Dr. Broadrick's response will cheer the most insurance-weary soul. Incidentally, although the insurance company never replied to Dr. Broadrick's letter, it paid the claim, no questions asked.—Ed.

The Insurance Company Writes . . .

Dear Dr. Broadrick,

We are reviewing a Major Medical Expense claim for the above-named patient. To determine the benefits available for your services, we need additional information and would appreciate your response to the following items.

1. What symptoms or problems did the patient report upon initial examination? Please be specific.
2. Please provide the details of your clinical findings, including range of motion, areas of pain elicitation and muscle palpation test.
3. Please forward to us the patient's pre- and postoperative X-rays, and additional diagnostic imaging reports and study models, if any. These will be handled carefully and returned promptly upon completion of our review.
4. Detail the proposed treatment plan, including your specific therapeutic goals and expected treatment frequency and duration.
5. If the treatment plan includes the use of an appliance, please complete the following:
   a. Does the appliance have a specific name, other than that describing its function? If so, please give the name.
   b. Does the appliance cover the *occlusal* surfaces of the teeth?
   c. Will the appliance protect the teeth from grinding, or reduce bruxing?
   d. Will the appliance move the teeth or change the occlusion in any way? Please describe.
   e. Is the appliance fixed (cemented in place) or removable?
   f. When (time of day or night) is the appliance worn? For what length of time will it be worn? How often will the appliance require adjustment?

We would appreciate your response as soon as possible since benefits are pending your reply. An authorization for release of this information is enclosed.

Kelly St. Jean
Claims Examiner

Dr. Broadrick Replies . . .

Dear Ms. St. Jean:

In response to your letter dated Dec. 30, 1993, and mailed Jan. 11, 1994, you must know my only contract and first obligation is to my patient, Mr. Bailey. I thoroughly explained to Mr. Bailey the how, why and need to have his bite equilibrated.

Your letter appears to be a ploy to either delay or avoid the benefits due Mr. Bailey. Before I spend the necessary time and added expense to answer all your questions, I need some information from you.

1. Please send the name of your dental consultant who will be reviewing the information you request.
2. Consultant's background:
   a. Dental school attended, year of graduation.
   b. List all courses taken in occlusion since graduation. When and by whom?
   c. Years of experience doing occlusal equilibration.
   d. Method of equilibration he/she advocates:
      —Pankey-Dawson
      —Myomonitor
      —Gnathology
      —Other—if other, explain.
3. Please explain how, by looking at before and after x-rays, your consultant can determine the need for occlusal equilibration.
4. Please have your dental consultant list all of the

*Reprinted with permission from *GDA ACTION*, The Journal of the Georgia Dental Association, May 1994.

necessary criteria that he/she uses to determine the need for occlusal equilibration. Be specific.

5. Please tell me the normal fee your company pays for complete occlusal equilibration.
   a. Does having 30 years experience doing occlusal equilibration have any bearing on the fee allowed?
   b. Please explain in detail how you arrive at a fair fee for occlusal equilibration.
   c. Explain how you plan to compensate me for the time spent now, and later, by answering your questions and providing x-rays and study models.
   d. Do you desire study models mounted on a functional, semi-adjustable articulator?

I would appreciate your response as soon as possible since Mr. Bailey's benefits are pending your reply. Please be specific and answer all questions.

Lawson K. Broadrick, D.D.S.

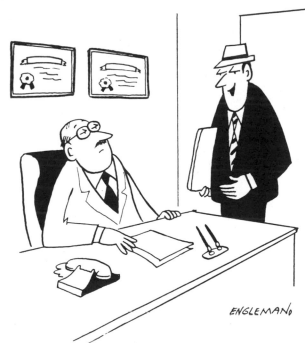

"It will help with office expense if you install a video game in your waiting room."

J. Engleman*

*Reprinted with permission from *Tic*, (May):15, 1989.

THERE'S MORE FOR YOUR LIFE AT YOUR DENTIST'S OFFICE*

Donald F. Bowers, D.D.S.

The idea of department store dental clinics bothers me. The basis of this feeling is neither one of legality or morality. It's more a question of image. Dental care at Sears? Come on, now. Dentistry doesn't belong in department stores with lawn mowers, DieHard batteries, refrigerators and clothing. I can barely accept the idea of buying automobile insurance in a department store. But dental care? Never. How can you practice dentistry in a place that has a candy counter?

It probably wouldn't do any good to ask the Sears, Roebuck Co. to get out of the dental clinic business. Apparently, there is money to be made from the operation. Otherwise, they wouldn't do it.

I could personally boycott their local stores in protest, but where would I buy Craftsman tools and Arnie short-sleeve, button-down, oxford cloth shirts? I could call on my colleagues who share my feelings to form a group boycott, but that could lead to difficulties with the Federal Trade Commission and the courts. I'm not about to go to jail over an issue of image.

How about competing with them? It's a free market and we're all patriotic Americans. That's one way to get their attention.

If they are going to sell dental services in their stores, dentists will sell merchandise in their offices. The dental offices wouldn't carry inventories of goods, of course. The purchases would be made at computer terminals placed in the waiting rooms. Private practice dentists would compete with Sears' catalogue sales. Here is how it would work.

The for-profit subsidiary of the American Dental Association could purchase merchandise from wholesalers in Taiwan, Korea and Yugoslavia which would then be stored in a warehouse in some central location like Topeka, Kansas. If the ADA can own buildings in Chicago and Washington, D.C., why not a warehouse in Topeka, for gosh sakes?

Dentists would buy computer terminals from the ADA which would be linked to the main computer in Chicago. The terminals would provide the customer or patient the current inventory of goods in Topeka with unit prices. The customer/patient could order directly through a terminal, purchasing goods like Dentmore washers and dryers at prices below those offered by Sears.

Customer/patients would be given a beeper when they enter the dental office. At anytime during treatment when a terminal becomes available, the beeper would signal the customer/patient who would leave the chair to go and buy things. Each office would receive a percentage of the profit.

Could the private practice dentists compete successfully? I think so. For one thing, Sears is only 100 years old and the profession of dentistry has been around since 1840. Also, there are more dental offices than Sears outlets. In Ohio, for example, there are around 4,000 or so dental offices and less than 50 Sears stores.

Marketing would be important. The dentists would need to place TV spots that out-class Sears' Pearle Dental ads. That shouldn't be difficult. Anybody would be better than Carole Whatsherface from the old Bob Newhart show. Why even the old Rivere clinic ad featured Pat O'Brien. How about a family-oriented commercial with Farrah Fawcett and Ryan O'Neill?

*Reprinted with permission from the *Ohio Dental Journal,* (Spring): 5, 1986.

LESSONS IN PRACTICE MANAGEMENT

TEMPORARY DRESSINGS*

Stephen Hancocks, B.D.S., L.D.S., D.D.P.H., M.C.C.D., R.C.S.

In the old days, a long white coat was all that was required, but nowadays your choice in surgery-wear says more about you than a packet of bleach ever did.—Ed.

In the same way that the abolition of school uniforms throws up tricky questions as to what children should be allowed to wear, so too does the modern trend in choosing what to wear in the surgery. Just like school uniforms or any other uniform for that matter, de-regulation comes as something of a mixed blessing. Certainly it is possible to indulge in self-expression of the garment variety, but with the attendant disadvantages that decisions have to be made. After all, if you can say it with flowers what kind of essay can you write with your wardrobe?

Style, colour, nuance, personality and the interpretation of mood all have to be considered and are, frankly, all PhD subjects in their own right which one ignores at one's peril. For the novice these are uncharted waters indeed. There are plenty of workwear catalogues to help with the choices, except that the greater the choice, the greater the confusion. We need to start somewhere though, so let us begin with style.

The starchy white, knee-length, patch pocket coat is definitely now only for fish fryers. So, it looks like it has to be an investment in a little waist level number, but with fastenings straight down or those shoulder buttons which, caught in a particular light, look just like a 'Torchy' puppet or a 'Joe 90' outfit?

Alternatively, one can take a rather more radical approach. Why not contemplate an all-in-one type of ski-suit affair with natty belt knotted casually, yet with the merest touch of professionalism, about the midriff. Not quite 'you' perhaps. Well you should not feel too left out for there is a school of thought which, rightly or wrongly, equates such apparel with Swedish garage mechanics (although always worth bearing in mind should your Volvo break down during a holiday in Uppsala). There are advocates, admittedly few and far between, of more extreme departures still. Shell suits, for example: how much closer to the people can one come? What price incandescent equality and what greater health and safety argument for making the patient wear protective glasses?

Which brings us neatly to colour. White? Too clinical or perhaps not clinical enough with cross-infection control to consider. Purity is everything. Or perhaps a blue, pastel being de rigueur and probably at the duck-egg end of the range. However, why stop there? The spectrum awaits from red through to violet, only the washing powder you use can intervene.

Footwear can be a problem. The starched longcoat required a certain conservatism, a pair of black leather Oxfords for example, or perhaps cheeky brown brogues for the country set. Sturdy, too, for those long hours spent on the hoof in the days when placing the patient supine still meant simultaneously dialing 999 and asking for the ambulance. Now, as with the clothing, the range is irritatingly open. Shoes still, but should they be slip-ons or tie ups? Clogs seem to be making inroads—however, these are definitely less advisable for practices on more than one level and where the clog wearers are destined to spend their days clumping up and down stairs. Also there are some rather alarming-looking boots putting in an appearance but one suspects that they must give a bet-

*Reprinted with permission from the British Dental Journal, 174 (7):256, 1993. This and the following paper also appear in a collection of columns by Dr. Hancocks, entitled *Do You Want to Spit in My Turnups or Dribble in My Basin?: An Anthology of Dental Humour*, published by the British Dental Association, London.

ter Harley-Davidson style sensitivity on the air rotor foot control.

All in all the array is bewildering, and it can easily make one start to yearn again for school uniforms. Surely other professions are not faced with such dilemmas; vicars, for example—a bible black shirt front and white dog collar, what could be more identifiable—and simple? But, for the dedicated image-changer the decisions are not over yet, since there is the rest of the practice team to consider. Should we 'team' the team, creating a double garage of Swedish mechanics, a practice of pastel pastiche? Skirts or trousers, co-ordinates or separates, contrasts or complementaries, and should there be a change week by week or should things always stay the same.

Finally, alarming as it may seem, one also has to consider how to start the consultation process. From the smallest to the largest practice, everyone is going to want to have their say and everyone will have their own particular very good idea. It does not really bear thinking about but do you remember the trouble we had with the logo? Well that was absolute child's play in comparison to the shifting quicksand on which the choice of work-wear is based.

Although that does also provide one further option—use of the practice logo on the clothing. All the same colour, all the same style and with the corporate badge of identity. Now that does begin to sound promising. Thank goodness we ditched that old uniform idea!

THAT VACANT LOOK*

Stephen Hancocks, B.D.S., L.D.S., D.D.P.H., M.C.C.D., R.C.S.

Archaeologists delight in discovering ancient dustbins and waste tips because of the valuable information that can be gleaned about day-to-day life. Classified job adverts fulfill a similar function.—Ed.

One of the most difficult and worrisome aspects of practice is finding the right person for the job, or conversely, finding the right job. The search often begins with the classified adverts in the *BDJ*, the nearest the dental profession gets to the equivalent of a fortnightly, employment, car boot sale.

It is the setting out of the stall which is so fascinating, just as the archaeologists can draw conclusions from the minutiae of medieval recycling sites, so too is it possible to create pictures of practices, and the often unconscious priorities of those who place adverts, from the contents of the copy.

Logically, three elements are involved—details of the job on offer, the location of the practice, and the most suitable type of person. However, the order in which they are stated is very revealing. Some adverts concentrate solely on the practice: 'Associate wanted for busy practice, full book, preventive-orientated, full support staff, immediate start.'

Indeed, some are so fulsome in their description that one wonders if they've bought the column space just for an ego trip. 'Delightful family practice in rural surroundings, full chairside and administrative support including hygienist and fully qualified DSAs, computerised, OPG, full clinical freedom, air conditioned, newly-equipped surgeries, laboratory on premises, intra- and extra-oral video systems, laser, fibre optic equipment, caring environment, VT registered . . .' One almost expects the last line to read, 'Not bad eh? All achieved from sheer hard work, determination and effort, and that from someone who didn't even go to public school . . .'

As with any advertising there is also the temptation to embroider the truth just a little bit, as in de-scribing the practice location. Indeed there are times when principals delve into the vocabulary of the estate agent: 'Delightful cathedral city,' 'Tranquil county town,' or, the slightly more suspicious, 'city centre practice with views to open ground on one side.'

Then again there is an alternative approach which involves the proximity of the practice to various transportation systems. Initially one might suppose that this is an indication of how easily patients can attend the surgery, but closer reading sows some seeds of doubt. 'Close to M25,' seems alright but the more mysterious, 'only 20 minutes from exit 4, M17,' begs the question as to whether this has more to do with a speedy getaway, as indeed does, 'channel ports within easy fast drive.' Of course such directions also leave a wide margin of imagination: 'only 10 minutes from Leeds,' fails to inform the reader as to what mode of travel is being quoted—foot, Porsche, Concorde, or perhaps air rotor. Even more rare is the recent, modest text which added, 'only 5 minutes walk from tube.'

Appealing to a certain type of potential colleague taxes the creative juices mightily. Constrained by the fact that partners, of the live-in type as distinct from the practice type, could also read the adverts, one suspects that the real personal details cannot be sent for typesetting. 'Curvaceous blonde with high IQ, good dress sense and excellent clinical skills,' may be desirable but what would the wife say? Similarly, in this age of sexual equality, 'Hunky, gym-training, Chippendale lookalike with interest in periodontology required for busy independent practice,' could err on the side of slightly questionable ethics.

*Reprinted with permission from the British Dental Journal, (Mar 5):195, 1994. This and the previous paper also appear in a collection of columns by Dr. Hancocks, entitled *Do You Want to Spit in My Turnups or Dribble in My Basin?: An Anthology of Dental Humour,* published by the British Dental Association, London.

LESSONS IN PRACTICE MANAGEMENT

Not that advertisers are slow to state ethical requirements, even if these might be expected to go, or arrive, without saying. Once again a notion of the type of practice can be surmised from the anticipated applicant. 'Experienced associate capable of high gross,' is hardly written to encourage the new graduate, while the only slightly less thrusting, 'fast energetic practice enhancer,' isn't exactly the signal for a diffident first-timer either.

Reasons for the need of a replacement are often not given. Retirement is mentioned, as is the fact that the dentist is leaving to start a family, take a course or work abroad. One has to assume that the phrase, 'needed to replace an *outgoing* colleague,' means the same thing, rather than that the surgeon in question was a manic exhibitionist.

Despite all the pretence there is probably no surer way to the potential responder's heart than the column inches which show the clearest sense of priorities, by alluding to dentistry as a means to an end. For example, 'Practice with much to offer new associate; sailing, excellent local properties at reasonable prices, good schools, rural walks, multitude of country pubs and first class restaurants, opportunities for gliding, sub-aqua diving, equestrian pursuits and windsurfing. Knowledge of dentistry an advantage. Morning sessions only,' would, one suspects, clinch it for most applicants.

WEATHERING THE PATIENT MANAGEMENT MONSOON*

Almost Everything a Senior Dental Student or the Newly Graduated Dentist, or, for That Matter, any Dentist Needs to Know to Remain Afloat

Paul Sassone

Has this ever happened in your office?

A patient arrives for his appointment. But as soon as he enters the waiting room, he suddenly feels better: "It doesn't (arrgh!) hurt so much (owww!) now, I think I'll (iieee!) come back (urggg!) some other time (yowww!)."

The reason is simple—your patient is afraid. In fact, your patient is an odontophobic.

About one-third of all people who visit a dentist do so because they are in pain. But the excruciating agony of an impacted third molar doesn't seem so bad to an odontophobic when he or she is faced with dentistry. Between five and six percent of the U.S. population avoid dental care because of fear.

Abandon Hope

For the dental team, fear is as great an enemy as caries.

Fear walks right into the waiting room with the patient. And so it is in the waiting room that fear must be dealt with.

It stands to reason that the waiting room should be a pleasant place to be instead of the waiting room to hell.

Here are some tips:

- Even if Dante is your favorite poet, it is a good idea not to have inscribed above your door, "Abandon all hope, ye who enter here."
- If the waiting room has a television, make sure movies such as "Marathon Man," or any other films that portray dentists as psychotic killers, are not shown.

- The right kind of piped-in music can soothe a patient in pain, but steer clear of heavy metal, the "1812 Overture," or any music that simulates the throb of a toothache.

Once the patient is inside the office, you, or if you are more established, your receptionist-cum-assistant, should greet the patient pleasantly—something between, "Well?, What?" and "Oooh, got a bad owie in your toofums?" will do nicely. (If you have a staff, you can skip this part and go on to the next section, although you might find it amusing.)

Ideally, you should check the patient's chart, know his or her name, and be aware of the problem so that even new patients can be greeted like old friends.

Patients shouldn't have to wait, but they do. There should be an ample supply of current, interesting magazines close at hand. You want to take the patient's mind off pain, so scientific publications with graphic illustrations of the latest in radical cancer treatment are probably inappropriate.

Give the patient an idea of how long he or she will have to wait. "The doctor will see you when he is good and ready," does not strike the right tone.

Time permitting (and if you are just starting out, you probably have plenty of time), engage the patient in some friendly chit-chat. Avoid questions for which the answer is yes or no ("Are you afraid to die?" is such a question). Ask about the patient's hobby (and hope it's legal) or the patient's family (and hope they're not all locked in a civil suit over Aunt Mamie's will). Just make sure the topic is something the patient is able to discuss. For example, "What do you think of Newton's Second Law of Thermodynamics" is probably a bad question.

By now the patient should be putty in your hands.

*Reprinted with permission from the *CDS Review*, 84(9):28–31, 1991.

Cover All Sharp Objects

Patients afraid of dentistry will not be put at ease by a glittering tray of your armamentarium. Keep your instruments wrapped in their sterile packets if you want to avoid answering the patient's anguished question, "Omigod! Are you going to use those on me?"

Make sure the patient is comfortably seated in the operatory chair before you tilt it back. Continue chatting about inconsequential topics as you/your staff unwrap the packets and don your/their protective gloves, masks and eyewear. Avoid such questions as "So, what's your greatest fear? Being eaten by rats or being buried alive?"

And now, for those who are staffed, it's time for the doctor to make his or her appearance. If your patients like your staff, they had better love you. The most common reason for a positive response to dentistry is a personal liking for the dentist.

"Good grief, your mouth looks like the Okeefenokee Swamp! When's the last time you were here, the Crimean War?" is not a good opening gambit.

Explain the procedure to the patient in layman's terms. Be pleasant, even jocular, but remember the patient is anxious if not downright fearful. He or she may not think that, "This is going to hurt you more than it will hurt me," is so hilarious.

The rest is just good dentistry. With patient handling, even the most fearful dental patients can be taught to relax in the dental office, thus freeing them to concentrate on other phobias.

And Now a Word from the Sponsor

Okay, you've done a good day's work. You've provided the best care you know how to provide and you've made your patients love you for doing it. Now comes the hard part: the bill.

This is a delicate area. It sometimes takes as much skill to deal with an impacted bill as it does an impacted third molar.

Never, never discuss a patient's outstanding balance in front of others. People in pain (or out of pain) are particularly touchy about being publicly embarrassed.

As a rule, discuss your fees and the method of payment with your patients in private and before beginning major treatment. Remember, you cannot threaten to replace an extracted tooth nor can you threaten to withhold anesthetic unless the patient pays the bill. Once you've communicated your fee and agreed on the method of payment, put it writing. And that should be the end of that—unless your patient has insurance.

Many good patient-dentist relationships have floundered on that one word: "insurance."

That's because, as we all know, the objective of insurance companies is to collect as much money as possible while paying out as little as possible.

With that objective in mind, insurance companies have invented the concept of "usual, customary and reasonable (UCR) fee." This is where the insurance company decides how much each dental procedure should cost.

To establish the UCR, insurance companies conduct a fee survey in Peru (or some other Third World nation), divide the average Peruvian fee by 12 and then deduct $14 to cover the cost of providing dentistry during a total eclipse of the sun. The total is what insurance companies are willing to pay for dental procedures provided in large US cities.

Unfortunately, the insurance-company-mandated UCR rarely bears any resemblance to a usual and customary fee in this area (and possibly in this solar system). But the patient doesn't understand this. Like the rest of us, he believes that everything costs too much these days, so he leaps to the conclusion that your fees are higher than the fees of any dentist in the world.

Don't take it personally should your patient question your integrity, veracity, or parentage. The patient just doesn't want to get stuck paying for something he thought he had insurance for in the first place.

This is another one of those times for a private conversation—actually this chat should have taken place long before treatment began. All you can do is try to explain the difference between the UCR and your fees and rely on the good relationship you have built by being kind, compassionate, amusing and understanding.

It's a delicate operation, not unlike the delicate dental procedures that you are good at.

MY LIFE IN NILAM*

David J. Pippin, D.D.S.

A new dentist buys a practice in an enchanting, small, rural town. . . .—Ed.

When I graduated from dental school that lovely spring day in 1978, my vision was fixed squarely on the future and on the student loans hanging over my head like dark and ominous clouds. I was eager and excited about embarking on my new career, anxious to tread the rosy path of setting up my own practice. The question, of course, was where? All of the large cities were full—over full, in fact. And, thanks to capitation and the helpful federal government, so were the medium-sized towns. That, I supposed, left only the small towns.

A quick glance through the ADA journal spotlighted this ad: "For sale. Modern office in lovely small town. Practitioner retiring. Will help finance." A drive in the country to that utopian hamlet, the future environs for my comprehensive oral health care services, was in order.

Four hours and a blinding rainstorm later, I was completely, totally, and inextricably lost. But up ahead was a street light, actually *the* street light—there was only one—in the peaceful, rural (very rural), pastoral town of Nilam. As the black rain clouds parted to reveal a glorious sunset over gently rolling meadows and fields, I knew. This was it.

With a bit of local help at the town square, I found the dental office. I introduced myself to the dentist and, after a bit of bargaining and a visit to the banker across the street, found myself gazing around my new office. Yes, the carpet was a bit tattered. And there weren't any windows, it was true. The chairs, for stand-up dentistry only, were completely manual. The drill was an antique belt-driven jackrabbit. (I had never actually seen one before, but I knew what it was.) Suction came from a wet/dry vacuum cleaner and a rather long rubber hose.

But the office did have one redeeming feature that endeared it to me above all others and more than made up for its shortcomings. It was mine.

The office also offered a bit of continuity—which I thought I needed to maintain rapport with the community—in the person of the office manager, Ruth. Ruth had run the office (well-chosen words) for the previous dentist for 45 years. Would she be receptive now to all the swell new ideas of this eager young graduate? Oh, sure. No problem.

I had already noticed several interesting things about the town of Nilam. For one thing, visitors could not get there by normal roads; they had to take a time machine. Going to Nilam was like stepping 50 years into the past. It was such a small community that on the dirt road leading into town was a hand-lettered sign reading "Entering Nilam," and on the back of the same sign was printed "Leaving Nilam."

The town was so small it had only one Yellow Page. I tried to call into town once, and the area code was busy. You had to make your own entertainment in Nilam, meaning that you planted your own garden and watched it grow. The only restaurant in town was an "all-night" diner that closed at 10:00 p.m. . . . The street light over Main St. was a bare 60-watt bulb, and if you plugged in your electric razor, the light dimmed slightly. The shopkeepers didn't have to take in the sidewalks every night in Nilam. The rain washed them away. The shopkeepers just put out fresh mud in the morning.

To enter the dental office, you had to go through a concealed side door in the common wall shared with the hardware store. There was no sign on the door, because, of course, everyone knew where the dentist's office was. Strangely enough, they really did! We had a lot of walk-ins—walk-in fillings and

*Reprinted with permission of the American Student Dental Association from *Dentistry87*, December 1987, pp 28–30.

extractions, that is. Folks would come in, sit in the chair, and point to the one that hurt.

A typical interaction might go like this: "It's the one in the back there with the hole in it, Doc. Never gave me any trouble before." Or: "It's the one that's broke back there, Doc. I was eating some mashed potatoes. . . ."

A quick look, an X-ray, and "You're in luck. I think we can save that tooth."

"How's that?"

"Well, just a little ol' filling back there and that tooth will be as good as new."

"A filling, huh? Won't that need replacing some-day?"

I would launch into my all-man-made-things-have-a-lifespan monologue.

"Naw, let's just git it out and be done with it."

"No, no. You don't understand. There are years of good chewing left on that tooth. It just needs a lit-tle filling." I often panicked at what they would ask me to do—tooth genocide.

"Nope. Let's just git it on out, and we won't have to worry about it no more."

In Nilam, I quickly learned, if you took out a tooth that was hurting, you were a hero. They really appreciated that kind of service. Slap you on the back, shake your hand, and call you friend. But if you saved that tooth with some kind of complex pinretained MODLXYZ amalgam—well, for one thing, they resented paying for something that would have to be replaced again someday, and, for another, you just might have taken food off the table that night.

People in Nilam thought of their teeth as little time bombs set in their mouth. They knew those lit-tle bombs were ticking away and would go off someday. The quicker they got them out the better. I spent many self-defeating hours trying to con-vince them to just maybe brush the fuses off. Tough place for a preventive program.

I got a lot of after-hours calls about toothaches, because—let's face it—why take time off work to go to the dentist when he would open his office at night for you? And the previous dentist had. For 45 years.

I still have to smile when I recall a certain 2:30 a.m. telephone call. . . . I had managed to incorpo-rate the persistent ringing of the phone into a dream I was having. In the dream, I was being unmerci-fully attacked by a giant, blood-thirsty mosquito that chased me deeper and deeper into a jungle of paperwork and dental floss. Just when he was about to sink his proboscis deep into my carotid, a flash of clarity revealed the real source of the ringing:

"Uh, hello?"

"Hello. Doc? Listen, I got this tooth that's just hurtin' somethin' awful. I can't stand it any more. Could you come up to your office and take it out for me?"

"Uh. Uh. What, what time is it?"

"Oh, about 2:30."

My head, just beginning to clear, chased away the last bits of sleep, and I asked perceptively, "a.m.?" I'm not at my best when I first wake up.

"(Chuckle) Yeah. I just got home."

Then I just had to ask, "How long has that tooth been hurting you?"

"Oh, about four weeks now."

Again, I just *had* to ask, "Why didn't you come in sooner?"

"I thought it might go away."

"Well," I said, "maybe it still will." Click.

But I guess it didn't, because he was sitting on my front steps at 8:00 the next morning, and I re-lieved him of that burdensome tooth.

My friend Joe owned the drugstore in Nilam. A comprehensive drugstore it was, too. Pharmacy, stationery, gifts, veterinary supplies, soda fountain. The only place left in America, a traveling salesman assured me, where you could still get a real straw-berry phosphate—and for only a quarter.

Unfortunately, Joe's fountain leaked. Dripped, rather, from one of the old-fashioned carbonated water nozzles. (The carbon dioxide tank was in the basement.) A nice, steady, metronomic drip that drove his wife nearly insane. As you might guess, soda fountain repairmen are not very plentiful nowadays. But finally, just to quell his wife's vocif-erous complaining, Joe found a plumber from the city to take on the task. I happened to wander in on the day he was attempting the repairs.

"See this washer?" the plumber asked Joe, hold-ing a small copper ring on his hefty and grimy fore-finger. "That's your problem. Doesn't seal any-more."

"Great. Fine. Replace it," said Joe barely glancing up from several prescriptions he was busily work-ing on for one of my patients.

"Can't. They haven't made these since about 1929. I'll have to put this one back in."

"Wait." The plumber had Joe's full attention now. "Go across the street to the hardware store and ask old Herman for one."

"No," the plumber laughed. "You don't understand. They haven't *made* these things since 1929."

"Trust me. Just go on over and ask."

The plumber turned away resignedly and walked out. The "Colonial Bread" screen door closed softly behind him. I chuckled as I watched him go. I had been in Herman's hardware store many times, and he had two of absolutely everything. You just couldn't believe how much merchandise there was in racks, bins, counters, hanging on the walls—and Herman knew where every single item was.

I didn't go with him, but I could picture the plumber walking in and holding up the washer, asking for a new one. Herman, staring at the washer flips through the cards in his 80-year mental inventory. "Oh, yes. Come along."

Herman goes to the back of the store, opens an old oak door and goes out into a small, faintly musty storeroom. Set in the ground is an ancient cellar door. C-R-E-A-K, the door is lifted back and the plumber peers down a set of wooden steps, as the dust settles. Down they go. A pull cord at the bottom of the steps lights a bare electric bulb that swings pendulously, casting odd canting shadows. Herman shuffles along the dirt floor peering into delapidated bins of merchandise. He bends down, reaches into a poorly lit cubicle, and pulls out a small, oily cardboard box. He blows the dust off the end and squints at the label, "Here, now. Can you read that? My eyes ain't so good anymore."

"J-68 size C," reads the plumber.

"Yep. That's it. How many did you want?"

"Just . . . one. How much?"

"Six cents." Herman had known years ago that Joe would need one of those someday, and in his mental file he ticked off one washer, J-68 size C, and replaced the box.

I found just as much to be in awe of in the other trades in Nilam. The banker was as friendly as a man could possibly be and as honest as the day was long. We kept counter checks from the bank in the dental office, and patients used them frequently. Banking procedures were predicated on the premise that people were honest, and, in Nilam, they were. Except, of course, for the few who weren't, but then, everybody knew who they were and made allowances for them.

The lawyer in town drew up wills, did people's income tax, handled real estate transactions and an odd assortment of other legal items. There really wasn't much else to do. People certainly didn't sue each other in Nilam. Wouldn't even have occurred to them to solve their problems in such a manner.

The other person in town with whom I had a fascination was the barber. He was a good one and had a nicely graduated selection of bowls by size. He could fit nearly any size head. Later I was to introduce him to alginate mixing bowls, which were more versatile and adapted much better to variously shaped heads.

I suppose all good things must come to an end. I remember my last day in Nilam. I was standing on the front porch of my rented house, watching the moving van try to negotiate the rutted dirt road, muddied by the previous evening's rain. As far as I could see there were fields, trees, rolling pastures, and grazing cattle. Definitely an idyllic scene. I could almost forgive the beasts their playful mooing all those long, dark nights when I was trying to sleep.

A cool wind rustled the leaves of the big cottonwood tree in the front yard, as if to wave good-bye. I turned to go, carrying with me happy memories of a simple time and innocent existence. The glitter of an associateship was pulling me back to the city, back to the future. . . .

HOW TO MAKE A MESS OF IT*

Betty Lee Kuhn, D.M.

Whether you plan to rent an office in a building or mall, or build from scratch in a new location, or just renovate and decorate your present office, there are a number of ways to make a complete mess of it.

These guidelines, if followed carefully, are guaranteed to help you blow the whole thing:

- Don't burden yourself with a lot of long-range planning. It's more fun to do things on the spur of the moment, even if most of them go wrong. A week ahead is time enough to begin major plans for your project.

- Before you buy any new office furniture, consider the alternatives. Maybe some of your friends and relatives have stuff they're about ready to throw away. Garage sales are often a fruitful source of unusual pieces. And if any of that won't match your new things, patients won't notice if you keep the reception room lights dim.

- There's no need to make a big production of purchasing new dental equipment. Why wear yourself out? Buy it over the phone. And if the salesman says there's a special group deal on sale, snap it up immediately. If the bargain you bought turns out to be assorted pieces in shades of burnt umber and sour-grape green, you'll have a color combination people will never be able to forget—no matter how hard they try.

- "Consider function before form when you buy," say the management advisors. Ignore it. If you like the looks of something, go ahead and buy it. Later, if you find it won't work with your new setup, think of the pleasure you'll have looking at it.

- If you're planning to relocate, it's now time to choose the geographic location. Don't waste your time and gas inspecting dozens of places. Just tell a real estate agent what you want, and he'll bring you a large collection of lovely pictures to choose from.

- He who hesitates is lost, so decide fast. Delay will only confuse you. The best rule is to follow your first hunch, please yourself, and forget all the stodgy rules and dull technicalities. For example, if you're a New York orthodontist, tired of the noisy city rat race, why shouldn't you relocate in that lovely wooded area upstate? Of course, when you finally inspect your new office site, you may find your nearest neighbors are a convent of nuns, ten miles away. But then, you got what you asked for—a lot of peace and quiet out in the middle of nowhere.

- Floor plans and precise measurements of the new office space needn't bother you either. If you're building or renovating, let the architect worry about them. And if you're moving to a rented space, you can always measure areas the day you move. Granted, there may be some of your furniture and equipment which won't go through doorways or fit into rooms, but it doesn't take long to tear down a few doors and a wall.

- If you're moving to a new location, keep overhead down and don't plan on more space than you're now using. One way you can skimp on space is by making rooms serve double duty. For instance, if you want to start a new preventive program, why go to the expense of a separate room for it? Use the bathroom for all patient education. It already has a comfortable seat and makes a fine control room for the patient who's in it (and also for those outside who can't get in.) A neatly printed time schedule on the door, warning patients when the room is tied up, should eliminate conflicting traffic jams.

*Reprinted with permission from *Dental Management*, 15(10): 95–97, 1975.

- Traffic patterns are another hangup for the nit-picking experts. Somehow, patients always manage to find their way from one room to another. So what if they must walk through the operatory to get to the bathroom. Listening for the toilet to flush can become a fun game for you. And for the patient in the chair, the sound of running water will have a tranquilizing effect.

- Keep away from the site where your office is being built or renovated. And don't interfere as the work progresses. Carpenters, plumbers, and electricians resent outside opinions or suggestions. Remember that you are only the dentist who will have to work there when they finish, so don't make a nuisance of yourself.

- Never let anybody talk you into foolish extras, like more plumbing, electrical outlets or soundproofing. After all, there's no reason why you have to have hot and cold running water in the lab, just because every other dentist does. As for soundproofing, suppose an occasional scream from the operatory can be heard by patients in the reception room? It will provide an interesting distraction and help them forget their troubles as they leave your office on the veritable run.

- Remember that designing and decorating is supposed to be fun. Keep it that way by excluding your accountant and keeping your plans secret from your business manager. With all his budgets and financial statements, he'll just throw cold water on your enthusiasm. This way you can enjoy buying everything you want all at once, then telling him about it later—if he's still there.

- You don't need an attorney either. What for? All you're doing is fixing up your office. You're a well-educated dentist, and you know all about lease options, maintenance responsibility clauses, contract bids, zoning laws and internal construction liability.

- Please yourself and forget about the patients. If you've always had a yen for gold velvet chairs, go ahead and buy them for your reception room. It's now or never and you deserve to get what you want. Just because you're a pedodontist, for example, doesn't mean you must lead a life of frustration. If you want antiques and other dentists try to discourage you, they're just a jealous group trying to make a carbon copy of you. Forge ahead with your original plans. If you explain to the children that the chairs are antiques, you can rest assured that your little patients will always remember, and will give them gentle care.

- The white carpeting, which is your last major installation, can be laid after your start back to work. The waiting patients can help the carpet layers, and they'll get through faster, thus saving you money.

The final touches make your office truly unique. And no matter who helps you with the rest of your decor, these final artistic elements in the reception room should be yours alone. They are authentic extensions of your personality, blending appropriately with what you've already done to the office.

Colorful paintings for the walls are a must. Since you're a rugged individualist, doing your own thing, here are a few you might want to consider: "The Bullfighter's Death," "London during the Black Plague," or perhaps that grand old 1730 favorite, "Extraction Without Anesthetic."

If you're a traveler, some of your souvenirs can give your office the personal touch. You might want to copy the globe-trotting dentist who decorated every room of his office with unusual items bagged or bought during his trips. For instance, from his jungle safari, he cleverly coordinated two matched shrunken heads, making an unforgettable lamp for his reception room. In the operatory, a coiled python, stuffed and mounted, became an eye-catching frame for the wall clock. And from his vacation in France, he brought back a small guillotine which he installed in his business office. According to him, it was a great success, because he never had another collection problem.

Of course, he never had another patient, either.

ODE TO A DENTAL HYGIENIST

(And a Few Others)

The "Dental Team." How many times have you heard that? Some practices even wear matching uniforms bearing tooth logos. The fact is, our success depends on others: front desk personnel, assistants, technicians, and hygienists. Think of what practice would be like without support staff! On the other hand, personnel management (aka refereeing) is among the most challenging aspects of practice.

ODE TO A DENTAL HYGIENIST*

Earnest Albert Hooton

This "Ode to a Dental Hygienist" was given by Earnest Albert Hooton, Harvard professor of anthropology, as the peroration of his address to the graduating class of dental hygienists at the Forsyth Dental Infirmary in July 1942.—Ed.

Hygienist, in your dental chair
I sit without a single care,
Except when tickled by your hair.
I know that when you grab the drills
I need not fear the pain that kills.
You merely make my molars clean
With pumice doped with wintergreen.
So I lean back in calm reflection,
With close-up views of your complexion,
And taste the flavor of your thumbs
While you massage my flabby gums.
To me no woman can be smarter
Than she who scales away my tartar,
And none more fitted for my bride
Than one who knows me from inside.
At least as far as she has gotten
She sees how much of me is rotten.

*Reprinted with permission from Foley GPH: *Foley's Footnotes.*
Wallingford, PA, Washington Square East Publ., 1972, p 125.

MIGRAINE*

Dr. Richard Galeone

Venus Jones, my new dental assistant, arrives for work on her first day with a trash bag full of pictures, powders, potions, pills, a small pistol, and an ear the size and color of a pomegranate. No one mentions the ear, for several of us suffer from chronic swellings of various anatomical parts. I just thank God she's here. She throws the bag onto the sofa in the lounge.

"Look at my ear," she cries, as if anyone can look at anything else. "Something must have bit me in the middle of the night."

Well, I think it had to be a werewolf or at least a copperhead, and I worry that the sight of this succulent peduncled from the side of her head will frighten the children and offend the normal-eared parents.

But enough already. I have high expectations of Venus Jones for she has been chosen from scores of qualified candidates who left messages on the *Philadelphia Inquirer's* answering machine.

"I never worked for a dentist before, but my sister-in-law cleans for a chiropractor and she says I'd be perfect for the job" . . . "My cousin, Sylvia, is a hygienist, and I like the sight of blood" . . . "I am currently an exotic dancer looking for a career change."

There is a fluttering of palpitations behind my sternum when I see, sitting in the chair, rocking to and fro, Lucinda, our first patient of the day and confirmed feces eater, whose dietary predilection once resulted in the cancellation of operating room time.

I was in the dressing room pulling on my scrubs when Dr. Chang, the anesthesiologist, came rushing in.

"I'm sorry, Rich," he said, "I can't intubate her on a full stomach."

Several witnesses in the surgical suite's holding area attested to Lucinda's having satisfied her hunger. And, although I do not share this morsel of history with Venus, I am less able to conceal the fact that Lucinda is also a screamer with alopecia vera, whose squealing attempts at escape conjure up visions of greased pig contests. The whole episode is very unfortunate, for I was hoping to impress Venus with the fact that she was joining a class practice, but I am rather afraid she misses that point as the visit ends with Venus having to throw her body across Lucinda's, while I, after whiffing Lucinda's breath, slip in a mouthprop and do a battlefield exam.

As Lucinda's flaccid body sways down the hall toward the reception area, Venus sags back against the wall apparently uninjured.

"Well," I say while fighting to control my respiratory rate, "that was interesting. I hope you're not discouraged." My dyspeptic smile assures Venus that Lucinda's having been scheduled first thing, first day is an aberration, an unhappy coincidence and the tightness in my chest begins to subside.

"My," says Venus. "My oh my." She is holding her head.

"What?" I say.

"I'm afraid I'm coming down with a migraine," she says. "My, oh my, oh my."

"Do you want an aspirin?"

"Won't help," she says. "Won't help at all. This just never happens any more. I'll need to fetch some bald peanuts. It's simply the only thing that helps. The only thing. Would it be too much . . . Could I run to the store? I'll only be a minute."

"By all means," I say. "After all, am I a brute who won't let an employee go the store? For bald peanuts? After working for more than an hour? On her first day? Of course she can go. I empathize with the problems of my employees. When they're in pain, I'm in pain. *Me casa, su casa*, and all that stuff. They're like family.

Forty-five minutes later Venus returns happily munching on a can of "boiled" peanuts.

"Try some," she says, holding the can under my nose. They are shelled and floating in a sea of brine. I take one and pop it in my mouth. It is slippery and

*Reprinted with permission from the *Pennsylvania Dental Journal*, (May/June): 43–44, 1994.

its texture is decomposed grasshopper belly. How do I know? I just do, that's all.

Just then, Mercedes, my other assistant, calls from room two.

"Dr. Galeone," she says, "can you get this separator in?"

Venus dutifully follows me into the other room.

"The mesial of the lower right six," says Mercedes.

When I was a child my father was interested in astronomy. On summer nights we would look at the stars through his telescope and he would tell me about Copernicus and Galileo and the projectiles that Wernher Von Braun was developing to take men to the moon. I cherish those memories and am distraught to realize that somewhere along the line I stopped thinking of rocket ships when I hear the word "projectile."

The light on little Annie's face is fully eclipsed by the shadow of an ear as I lean over to look in her mouth. She waits until there is no chance of error and then projectiles onto my face, into my mouth, up my nose and into Venus's hair. Mercedes throws herself out of the line of fire. Venus pukes on my neck and shoulder. Since you ask, it tasted almost as bad as that boiled peanut.

While Mercedes works with the high-speed suction slurping up spaghettios and making hickeys on my neck, Venus runs from the room yelling, "My, oh my, oh my, oh my," to find some towels. But she runs past the desk, picks up her bag of pills and powders and dashes from the office. Go figure.

But what the hey. Maybe I'll give that exotic dancer a call.

CALLING ALL TECHNICIANS!*

Robert E. Horseman, D.D.S.

The Golden Age of dentistry is not moribund or even slightly under the weather, according to those who have their fingers on the pulse. On the contrary, they exalt, the Golden Age is getting its second wind and the days ahead never looked more promising. Although I view such pronouncements with some skepticism, hey, it's what I need to believe! So in spite of some evidence to the contrary, I'm going along.

What I *really* want to hear is that some school called the Polytechnic College of Dental Maintenance has just graduated its largest class ever, some 9,652 qualified technicians and dental repairpersons, bringing the ratio of dentists-to-repairmen down to 2:1. That's what I want to hear, because I don't think any renaissance of the Golden Age is going to occur with the present ratio of 100,000:4. This crisis, which receives nowhere near the attention of the present auxiliary shortage, is a bit of a puzzlement considering that the average repairman can earn about ten times what the average new dental graduate can expect after eight years in graduate studies.

Try this. Pick up the phone right now and call the person you'd like to think of as your connection with the dental repair business. If he doesn't have an unlisted number, tell the person who answers—IF the phone is answered at all, it most certainly will not be the actual person who does the repairing—that you've lost all your compressed air and the vacuum system is shot too. Even if you have to leave your message after the sound of the beep, start counting to one hundred billion by ones. Now try this: give up.

So what I want to know, as we embrace all the wonderful techniques and equipment of the Cosmetic/Perio Age, is where are all the people well-versed in everything from A-dec to Zeza coming from? Does the College of Polytechnic Maintenance actually exist with campuses in every state?

Does it have football teams, sock hops, frat houses and sororities and school yells?

Onward men, right to the peak!
Grab that wrench, fix that leak!
Splice 'em, mend 'em, solder 'em too!
There's not a damn thing we can't do!

Well, I'm sorry. Maybe things will be better five or ten years down the road, but right now you're pretty much on your own. That's why I'm offering (as a public service, since no CE units have been approved by the California Board of Dental Examiners) the following information regarding those two vital pieces of dental equipment, THE COMPRESSOR and THE VACUUM SYSTEM.

Basically, the compressor is a machine which sends air off in one direction, and the vacuum is another machine which brings it all back again along with whatever disgusting things it can pick up along the way. At first blush, it would seem that one machine with a reversing switch on it would be the sensible way to go. And so it would, except for a bad decision made many years ago when it was mandated that both these activities had to go on at the same time, or as we came to call it, "simultaneously."

Many present-day dentists don't know this, but there was a time in the distant past when a primitive device known as a "saliva ejector" was the only source of vacuum that operators had. Although it was immensely popular with patients, many of whom still chuckle today recalling the keloid tissue which paved the floor of their mouths, dentists demanded, and finally got, enough suction to empty a five gallon bottle in three seconds and to defuzz the air conditioner ducts in five.

Early air compressors were a marvel of simplicity. The machine consisted of a rubber bulb (usually black) attached to a narrow curved tube of metal. When the clinician squeezed the bulb, air rushed out of the narrow tip. The beauty of the design was that when the operator released his squeeze, the machine became a vacuum device. Alas, like so many

*Reprinted with permission from the *Journal of the California Dental Association*, 18(4):79, 1990.

other inventions offered before their time, the bulb syringe fell into disuse when dentists demanded and got enough air to completely change the contents of the Holland Tunnel in 15 seconds flat.

Both the present-day air compressors and the current vacuum systems are so ugly and noisy that they must be positioned in the very furthest recesses of your building. Manufacturers of these machines, of course, will deny this, but you'll notice that no one in their right mind puts either unit in their operatories. Indeed, the things are often so remote, the dentist has never actually seen the compressor or vacuum, believing the services come from someplace like Hoover Dam. That is, until that fateful day when one or both machines, in a fit of pique, pack it in.

Although I am reluctant to subscribe to some current theories that machines have some kind of native intelligence (and a malevolent one at that), still, they do seem to behave at times as if revenge was the only thing on their check-list. An itinerant repairman explained it to me this way once: "The compressor, you see, serves primarily the head man, sending him nice, clean air. They have a good symbiotic relationship. The vacuum, on the other hand, serves a perceived underling, the assistant. Furthermore, the assistant shows no gratitude for the service, but sends back unspeakable things. The compressor, knowing this, lords it over the vacuum, causing it to have an inferiority complex. In time, the vacuum curls up in a fetal position, refuses nourishment and that's that."

Fortunately for us, both machines usually respond to a show of attention on your part, a little TLC, so here's what you do in case of function failure: Grab an eight pound sledge from your tool kit and go down into the bowels of wherever your machines lurk. Taking a firm, overlapping grip on the handle of the sledge, give the recalcitrant machine a couple of good healthy whaps on any surface that will not deflect the blows onto your kneecap. The machine should start right up into its old familiar *tapocketa-pocketa* rhythm. If it balks, whack it again until something breaks, then sit down and calculate the cost in money and aggravation of getting it fixed by you-know-who or buying a new one.

YUCATAN*

Dr. Richard Galeone

Sure, now I can see the problem was traveling *cognito*. And in retrospect I won't do it again. But let me get behind myself and return to Thursday, noonish, when I was in my operatory with a new patient and his young mother. The intercom crackled to life with the receptionist's voice.

"Dr. Galeone? There's a man says he's Robert Redford on the phone."

The mother's eyebrows rose.

"Bob?" I said, grabbing the phone.

"Dr. Galeone? Please don't be upset. It's Gunther."

"When will you be in town, Bob?"

"I want to talk to you about disability insurance," said Gunther.

"No. Really, Bob. No trouble at all," I said. "What? I'll have Lorena pick you up at the airport. See you on Saturday," I said and hung up.

So I had a little fun at Gunther's expense. Big deal. He was driving me insane. Every 12 minutes on the phone trying to sell me insurance. It's the Cardinal's office, the White House, Mother Theresa. Tell him I've been harassed out of my mind. Tell him I had a heart attack. Who do I call to collect disability? Just don't let him through tomorrow. I'm leaving for my seminar on Saturday.

So, it's Saturday morning and I'm sitting on the plane just as pleased as a puppy with two peeders. I'm big-boned so I have to suck hard to get the 40-inch belt around 50 inches of bellybone. The Aeromexico crew cha-chas on board yelling "Hey, baby" and "Oh, mama" and "Woofwoofwoofwoof" while working its way to the cockpit. El Capitan is 20-something and I try to remember the words of the Act of Contrition. But what's this? Another passenger? Yes. Behind the captain comes a man with a gold cigarette holder, pince-nez and a weasel's twitchy nose. Gunther!

I slump and pivot and burrow into my carry-on as Gunther's butt slides over my elbow. He doesn't see me but I have to hold my head askew as if I have a stiff neck. We rocket to cruising altitude and I hear an "Eeeeee-Haaaaa" come from the cockpit. Teenage stewardi break out tequila, real glasses, salted rims, ice cold. People who do not require aphrodisiac, slurp worms.

There is turbulence *ad infinitum*. I pop 10 mg of Dramamine. It gives me dry heaves in a paper bag and I hear Gunther telling jokes as I retch up the back end of my gastrointestinal tract. We plummet to the earth.

To Lorena's disgust I linger at the end of the line in customs. The humidity's not bad but it's a million degrees. People burst into flame. But not Gunther. No. He gets into an air-conditioned limo.

"Can we go now?" Lorena asks in her "I could have married an orthodonist" voice. She doesn't notice that we are driven to Cancun by a lunatic. Tires leave the ground as we careen around a corner at mach two. I look over and she's putting on lips. Cars blur by and to my horror, I see Gunther's face in her compact mirror. Our driver pulls over and asks me to check the tire. Ees there air in zee tire? Okee dokey. No tip. There will be NO TIP for this sleaze bag. NO TIP AT ALL. How ees dat, my fren? But I'm so elated to be alive when he dumps us at the hotel that I overtip.

We eat. We drink. We seminar. And three days later, we go on the optional tour to Chichen Itza. We gather in the early morning breeze of the bus' exhaust fumes. Rumors circulate about tourists shot by banditos the previous week. We squeeze into the seat, worm our way through Cancun streets and turn down a dirt road through forest.

Ten minutes into the trip, I notice an intestinal rumbling, a rumbling of rapidly-growing, peristaltic-crazed bacteria. Bacteria wildly intent on shortening and narrowing my agonized colon so that I will be humiliated before my dental colleagues who have taken the precautions of boiled water and antibiotic

*Reprinted with permission from the *Pennsylvania Dental Journal*, (Nov/Dec): 37–38, 1994.

prophylaxis. It is in the 11th minute that I do not discover a restroom on the bus.

In the 12th we reach cruising speed of 100 miles an hour and Señor the driver is not going to endanger our lives by stopping so that banditos can rob and kill us and he lose his job just because some gringo cannot hold it like a man. There will be facilities at the gift shop in Chichen Itza. I will just have to bounce merrily along for another 3 hours and 43 minutes.

"DR. GALEONE," calls a voice from behind.

No. Gunther? Is this some cruel joke? Has my whole life been nothing more than an autistic hallucination? Are those things I did in the '60's coming back to haunt me?

"I CAN'T BELIEVE IT. I'M HERE WITH A GROUP OF INSURANCE SALESMEN. IT MUST BE FATE. WHAT ARE THE CHANCES? I MEAN STATISTICALLY? WHAT WOULD THE TABLES SAY?"

They would say pick up the pieces of your broken life and mail them back to Pennsylvania. Am I having fun yet?

"WHATZA MATTER? AREN'T YOU GLAD TO SEE ME? YOU LOOK ALL SWEATY."

"Little touch of Montezuma. I'll be okay."

"YOU DIDN'T DRINK THE WATER, DID YOU? GEEZ, DON'T YOU EVEN KNOW THAT? HERE, TAKE SOME PEANUTS."

"No." And then mercifully, nausea begins to distract me from the cramp.

"Uh oh," says Gunther.

I look up and the bus slows to a stop. There is a tree across the road. Señor the driver takes two guns from a box by his seat, gives one to the tour guide, Miguel, and they go out to move the tree. No one speaks. Not even Gunther. We look out into the woods. Even the bacteria know. They go into reverse peristalsis. Quickly they move the tree. There is yelling. A shot is fired. The driver and Miguel run back to the bus. Miguel tells us to lay low and the bus groans forward.

We get there about a million years later. Lorena goes with the other dentists and their healthy wives up the crumbling pyramid of El Castillo while I sit crouched with Gunther on a rock equidistant from that pile of stone and the room called Hombre. His nose twitches with the heavy scent of money and he regales me with tales of the underinsured. I pray for mercy. My skin blisters under Yucatan's sun. He tells me of the happy day when he first made the million dollar club. Oh joy.

I seek refuge in one of Hombre's stalls. But from the next cubicle he tells me his is full service. I wonder at this, but then he's talking about life and accident and health and . . . the elastic of my shorts has eaten into burnt flesh and methane putrefaction is causing stretch marks across my abdomen. Somewhere in my delirium I submit. I sign blank forms and Gunther leaves me to die. The afternoon is spent in the stall and when finally I crawl out only the mosquitoes are happy to see me.

"I must be getting hungry," says Gunther after a while on the bus. "I feel a rumbling in my stomach."

HOW TO RELAX

For Better or for Worse*

Lynn Johnston

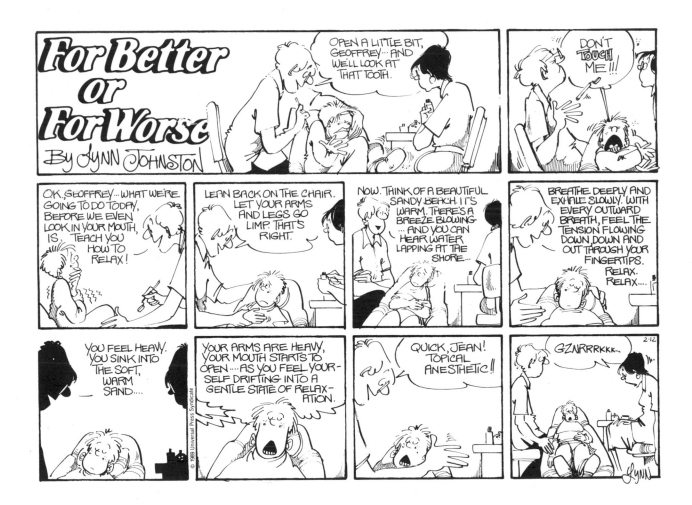

ODE TO A DENTAL HYGIENIST

LIFE BEYOND THE OPERATORY

Dentists, as a group, are individualists. Many are entrepreneurial. Practicing dentistry is hard work. And what would we do with more "free" time? These elements form the key ingredients for the pieces in this section. And what would we do with more "free" time?

A DENTIST'S GUIDE TO FITNESS*

Robert E. Horseman, D.D.S.

The human body. This God-given temple of the soul. Treasure it from birth, nourish it with oat bran and wheat germ, stoke it with vitamins and minerals, baste it with Oil of Olay, this marvelous machine. Give it a massage and aerobic exercises, treat it to Nautilus and every other body-enhancing gadget and potion from the fertile minds of man and Elizabeth Arden, then protect it from every kind of stress you can and you know what?—that sucker will die anyway.

It's ironic, like learning that Ponce de Leon, after years of searching for the Fountain of Youth, finally finds it just off I-95 and approaches the attendant for permission to bathe. "No problemo," says the Seminole-in-charge (sic), handing him a towel. "Fifty pesos and don't forget to take off your . . ."

But Ponce, eager to enjoy the fruits of eternal youth, jumps in still clad in his armor and plummets to the bottom like a safe.

Well, what did you expect? When you signed up for dental school, they didn't mention the nature of the work? C'mon, everybody knows about the postural and visual defects that set in about the second semester and go downhill from there. You didn't think for a minute, moron-like, that you were going to sit in a high-back leather chair issuing orders, giving dictation and doing three-martini lunches, did you?

No, it's our lot in life to give new meaning to the biblical phrase "laying on of hands." To do this requires that we get fit and remain so even if it means eventually questioning the validity of the whole concept.

Initiated by dentists still young and naive enough to think they could reverse this deterioration, the ongoing fitness craze that has gripped this country for the past couple decades shows no sign of abating. Orthopedic offices throughout the nation are littered with shin splints, torn tendons and sorely abused bodies. What we've got to do is sort out the things that will cripple or maim us, thus making us ex-dentists, and seek out those things that will give us a better

chance at fulfilling our destinies. The following information will not help a bit:

Right off the bat, so to speak, that eliminates baseball, as it is one of the sports invoking the use of hands, our most productive appendages, or at least the ones we're most interested in here. Lose the use of your hands and what's left for you?—nothing but the lecture circuit, a scam that's already been thought of by hundreds of your colleagues to the point where in a few years there will be nobody left to do the actual work; they're all be out lecturing to each other.

So let's see what might contribute to your fitness program without the danger of forcing you out to tell other dentists how to bleach teeth.

Golf

Golf gets you into the open air, and it's where patients think you are on Wednesdays anyway, but that's about all you can say for golf. To participate, it is necessary to humiliate yourself by wearing ridiculous pants and impractical shoes whose only other use is tenderizing cheaper cuts of meat. You sit on your dental stool, you sit in your golf cart. You try to get a small object into a hole, and you have a level of frustration as high or higher than in your practice. Golf does not contribute to your fitness but forces you to recite long, boring anecdotes whose tediousness is exceeded only by the tales of your fellow golfers.

Bowling

Forget bowling, too. Using three of your vital fingers to propel a large leaden sphere in an effort to flatten 10 objects just so you can do it again and again to the accompaniment of gawdawful noise makes no sense at all. The requisite costume is an embarrassment from the garish shoes to the sport shirts with embroidered advertising for brake relinings or fast food joints. Bowling would be bad enough if you did it alone, but tradition requires that you do it in concert with a bunch of bozos whose motivation is based entirely on getting a night out.

*Reprinted with permission of the *Journal of the California Dental Association*, 24(2):74, 1996.

Tennis

Tennis used to be a gentleman's game. From the crisp, white, impeccable outfits to the strict adherence to manners and tradition, it seemed to fulfil all the requirements. Even though the dominant forearm risked resembling Popeye's while the other one remained like Olive Oyl's, it was still a fairly civilized sport. This has changed. If you've watched any tennis lately, you know that Andre Agassi, with his sartorial statement, is now a role model; a tennis ball traveling at speeds in excess of 120 mph can alter your physical well-being forever; and there is way too much sweating and grunting. Umpires risk getting a biff in the snoot for a bad call, and people have been known to get stabbed. It became apparent just after the game was invented that running around in the hot sun chasing a little ball was a dumb thing to do. That's why the scoring was altered to jump from 1 to 15 to 40 just to get the game over with as fast as possible. Dentists are advised to take up pingpong, which is the adult version of tennis without the sun.

Scuba Diving

Younger dentists who miss the excitement of doing wheelies on a motorcycle with no hands, no helmet, and no brains or racing around in their father's Oldsmobile without benefit of functioning thought processes, frequently take up scuba diving as an antidote to the deadly confinement of the operatory.

Unless you live in Tahiti, Hawaii, the Bahamas or the Grand Caymans, you will experience only grinding regret every time you look into your closet at the jillions of dollars worth of wet suits, regulators, masks, fins, booties, hoods, gloves, depth gauges, tanks and special wrist watches the size of a manhole cover with 89 functions, none of which reveal the correct time, getting dusty from disuse. I realize that to a dedicated scuba diver this is all offset by the sight of a fish going by in its own element deep in the murky depths of water two degrees above freezing, but to a rational person, 30 minutes of a Jacques Cousteau rerun should suffice.

Skiing

You would think that a dentist, even a young one without the wisdom that comes from years of listening to patients lie about their flossing habits, would see the idiocy of falling totally out of control down the face of a mountain while wearing 7-foot boards strapped to boots the size of microwave ovens. Boards that he waxes to make him fall even faster, for God's sake. Well, lots of dentists do this. You can observe these dentists around the resort bars bemoaning their rotator cuffs and spiral fractures. It's the only sport open to dentists that requires more expensive gear than scuba diving. The cost of stuff needed for a family of four just to get to the falling-down stage of skiing exceeds that of the S&L bailouts. Skiing does not contribute to fitness, it cancels it.

Jogging

Nobody jogs anymore. I just put that in here so that if you are still jogging based on the misguided idea that it's doing you some good, you'll know it's time to quit. Power walking is where it's at now. With your $125 special cross-training walking shoes that has Korea giggling all the way to the bank, you'll discover power walking is to plain strolling what St. Vitus' dance is to Barcalounging. If you insist on power walking, do it in the early hours or after dark so that passing motorists won't lose control with laughter and crash into light poles.

That doesn't leave us with much. Certainly dentists with IQs superior to paramecia should eschew pumping iron. That branch of insanity will instantly identify any aneurysm you may have in your body, besides running the risk of making you appear to have had badly managed silicone injections inflicted on areas where you don't even have muscles and never did.

I know it's too late to save you from the mistake of buying the stationary bicycle, rowing machine, treadmill and the like. The only benefit these machines have ever produced accrued to the chuckling dealer who sold them to you. Leave them in the closet, under the bed with the dust bunnies or in the garage where they have resided peacefully since the second week they were brought home with such high hopes and firm resolutions.

Above all, don't be too hard on yourself for being such an incredible jerk for getting in such bad shape in the first place. And if you decide to take up one of these "fitness" sports in spite of all intelligence to the contrary, be sure to check with your physician before you start. You know what kind of great shape he's in.

THE PARENTING ADVANTAGES OF DENTISTS

The Far Side*

Gary Larson

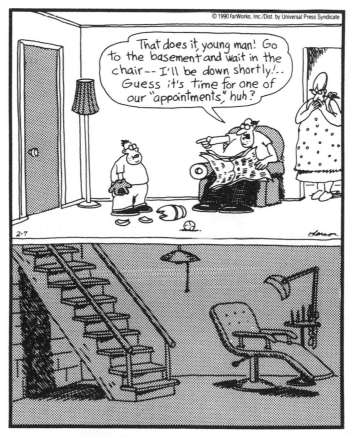

The parenting advantages of dentists.

CAMPO DENTISTA*

Dr. Richard Galeone

In days of yore, I spent many Saturday afternoons at the Mayfair Movies, where, for a dime, I saw cartoons and a double feature. So one may surmise of which yore I speak.

Inevitably, in one of those films, there would be a British soldier named Smithers who was mistakenly left for dead out in the desert. Then, dehydrating down to a beef jerky, he would slither for days toward the cool palms of an oasis only to discover it just a mirage. The camera would pan into the wind and drifting sands of the Sahara amidst the sound of hysterical laughter. One would hear a shot. Then, silence. I never grieved at any length for Smithers or gave much thought to the incompetents who left him out there to die until years later.

Campo Dentista is a boot camp where legions of dentists have assembled just west of the Red River at the foothills of the Wichita Mountains where tumbleweeds roll and cattle roam free. Big black beef cattle.

A drill sergeant nameth Roy "The Cow" Roykowski with a history of dry, high-speed unanesthetized cavity preparation is marching us through thorn and briar in egg-cooking heat. I wash down a salt tablet with the last few drops of iodized water. No one is sweating save Roykowski, who has brought three canteens and drinks from them freely, letting the excess waste over his chin. Great patches of sweat that look like the continental plates of Africa and South America grow together from his pits across the olive sea of his shirt.

He is droning on about the merits of honor and loyalty, about edible roots and how to cross a stream atop a fallen branch. Survival things. Manly things. He suggests we not wipe ourselves with poison ivy and when he's done, I tell him we're thirsty.

He grabs me by the trachea and pulls me from the line.

"Thirsty," he says, apparently horrified by my weakness. "This is what's wrong with America. This is why we're losing the war. You pansy. Isn't mommy here to take care of you?" (I believe this question to be rhetorical.) "What a marine," he says, even though we're in the Air Force. "What a credit to the corps. Does anyone here want to share his water with this?

No one moves.

He pushes me back towards the line with a parting epithet and I feel a dry bolus racing north in my esophagus. I swallow hard not to vomit.

Upon my return to camp, I find a can of tomato juice in a pack of World War II K-rations. Without injuring myself, I attack it with a Swiss Army knife. I am parched to clinical dementia. When I puncture the can, a volcanic puff of red spray spews forth and in the mist of that spray, I behold a vision of poor old Smithers dressed up in the garb of Saint Apollonia wielding Excalibur, and I hesitate. What is the meaning of this warning? Has some botulistic bacteria cultured within the can? No, it can't be. It is simply the east Texas heat and I lift the can to my lips.

But before that nectar reaches my mouth, Roykowski swoops down, grabs it, drains it with one gurgling suck and flies away. I feel (to my shame, really) like Hitler on six cups of coffee but internalize my homicidal tendencies for personality development.

And it comes to pass that later that night I am awakened for a mock emergency. I am designated a triage officer and after several decisions, I behold a fellow off in the high grass moaning to himself. He is doubled over and maketh really convincing retching sounds. As I approach, he doth whisper, "Get me to yon latrine."

To my dismay, I see a pale and clammy Roykowski. He says he feels like he's going to die. I say so what—to myself.

Our leader ails so mightily that he can no longer speak as I drag his carcass down the hill and over

*Reprinted with permission from the *Pennsylvania Dental Journal*, (May/June): 45–46, 1993.

the dirt path toward the eau de toilette of the latrine which is a rectangular tent with a flap at either end. Inside, six seats are lined up. No stalls. No privacy. Just six holes in the ground. I do not accompany him to the throne, but am able to fathom the rich pageantry of life unfolding within.

As Sergeant Roykowski feels his way to a seat through perfect darkness and, at long last, relaxes the sphincter that has protected his dignity, a trumpet blast sounds, which, by some bizarre twist, resembles the mating snort of an Angus cow. This is closely followed by a rumbling of the earth, a series of percussions resembling an aboriginal clicking language and, finally, a sulfuric gust which makes the tent flaps—well—flap.

It is at this moment that the anguished Roykowski beholds two dull red orbs hanging in the darkness just ten feet to the east. Then to my surprise, as well you may imagine, and in less than one minute subsequent to his crouched entrance dance, he sprints out of the western end of the tent at 60 miles an hour, which is all the more remarkable as his pants and shorts are gathered below the knees. And even more extraordinary, is the fact that close on his heels, in amorous pursuit, is an Angus bull with flaming red eyes in the full throes of his annual rut. It is not an exaggeration to say that I was shocked. Wow! For even though I had spent many a summer on my grandmother's chicken farm in New Jersey, I had never witnessed this level of interspecies attraction.

And behold, there once was a power of mystical origin that protected dentists against the forces of injustice. And woe be to him that lifts the sword against the toothsaver, for his bowels will be in an uproar and he will live with the beasts of creation. And it comes to pass that Sergeant Roy "The Cow" Roykowski is not released from the intensive care unit until after I am stationed at a SAC base in the remote forests of northern Maine, but I think of him with fond remembrance every time I see one of those old British war movies.

GETTING OUT OF DENTISTRY*

Donald F. Bowers, D.D.S.

I was excited a few weeks ago when I received an advertisement through the mail for a set of audio cassettes, prepared by one of my colleagues, designed to teach me how to get out of dentistry painlessly and into some other livelihood. It is timely in my case since I am on the verge of beginning my third mid-life crisis.

What prevented me from filling out the form and mailing it with my check for $385 was $385. That's a bit steep for one set of cassettes. I can get "The Big Hits of the '60s" for $10.95 plus mailing. Chuck Berry, Buddy Holly, the Supremes and the Beach Boys for $10.95? What could be worth $385?

Nonetheless, the advertisement set me into action. If I'm going to get out of dentistry, now's the time. Thirty years in this lousy profession and what's it gotten me? A nice home, a sense of financial security, the respect of my friends and neighbors, many grateful patients and a gold credit card through the ADA. It's not enough. I want glamour in my life. Dentistry is not glamorous, not exciting enough.

I contacted the Central Ohio Career Counseling Center which promised to help me select a new career for $125, which sounded more reasonable than the cost of the tapes. What's more, the Center provided personal one-on-one service. When I reported for my appointment, the lady at the desk smiled and greeted me.

"Mid-lifer, eh?" she asked. "Well, don't worry. We have some special counselors who are trained to work with you . . . ah . . . ah . . . ah, more mature clients."

"Swell," I said, eager to get started.

I spent four hours taking a battery of tests that included looking at inkblots and answering questions about everything. I was told to report the following week for the post-test interview.

The next day, I had lunch with an old high school buddy who is an attorney—mine, as a matter of fact.

I told him, "I'm getting out of dentistry. I'm tired of it and I want to do something glamorous and exciting."

"Like what?" he asked.

"Like being a lawyer," I offered. "It must be exciting pleading a case in front of a jury like Perry Mason or like Paul Newman in 'The Verdict'.

"Believe me, it's not," he said. "Courtrooms are a small part of the work and I don't find it exciting at all. Most of my day is spent trying to keep a bunch of angry, unhappy people from killing me or each other; the rest of it is a lot of dull busy work. Frankly, I'm thinking about getting out of law. I'm tired of being equated with ambulance chasers and Shylock. I've had it with shark jokes."

"What are you thinking about as a new career?" I asked impulsively.

"I'll tell you I don't know yet but if I were younger I would think about dentistry. People respect dentists and if you're nice to them and show them you care about them, they love you. People don't begrudge you your fee like they do a lawyer's."

The next week, I returned to the Career Center for my interview. The lady who was specially trained to work with the more mature clients was more mature herself. She told me she had been an air [traffic] controller before she went into psychology.

"Being an air controller must be exciting," I said, surprised that someone would want to do something less exciting.

"It's the pits," she informed me. "The President did me a big favor when he canned me."

She told me that they had carefully analyzed the tests I had taken, considering my interests, likes and dislikes, attitudes, and aptitudes.

"Your composite scores clearly indicate that you are suited for one occupation far above any other," she announced.

"And what would that be?" I asked breathlessly. "A jet pilot? Grand Prix race car driver? CIA agent?"

"Dentist," she said. "Unfortunately, you may be a little old to be thinking about dental school now. Too bad you didn't come here years ago. No question about it. You should have been a dentist."

"But I am a dentist," I told her, obviously irritated. "I want to do something else that's exciting and glamorous. That's why I came here."

"I understand," she claimed with a knowing smile. "There's only one problem. All of the occupations that are exciting or glamorous require you to stay up at night past 10:30."

*Reprinted with permission from the *Ohio Dental Journal*, (Fall):5–6, 1986.

HOW TO REALLY EARN $500,000 A YEAR IN DENTISTRY TODAY*

The big bucks are on the lecture circuit.

Richard B. Winters, D.D.S.

The only sure way to be fantastically successful in dentistry is not to do dentistry at all.

Instead, you can make all the money you'll ever need by presenting a course showing a unique, theoretical or practical technique applicable to clinical dental practice, or by evolving a new idea in the field of practice management. Yes, you too can ensure success through show and tell.

It seems, though, that everyone is giving courses today, so some guidelines and rules are in order.

The following do not have to be strictly adhered to. You can modify or abridge them to suit your tastes.

I. A Secret Word

This is a must. A new word or acronym must be emblazoned in capital letters in the literature advertising your course. Your secret word can be something like "successodontics" or "beer nuts." Find a secret word that you can really live with, not one that's inane and doesn't have any deep meaning.

In your course syllabus make sure that you don't use a word like "modality," which has been done to death. Only dentists have ever seen this word in print.

Your secret word can also be exotic—like "Yabdook." If Yabdook ever goes over, you can go to Yabdook II or III for a more select clientele at higher fees.

Acronyms are real eye-openers:
- EMM (Earn More Money)
- LWMP (Less Work More Profit)
- QUIP (Questing Universal Improved Practice/Profits)

II. The _____ Technique

If you have really done some terrific work that nobody knows about, you can call it the Lumpkin Technique—if your name is Lumpkin.

Everyone is into bonding—so that's out. Your technique must be quick, efficient, painless, and costly.

A real beauty could be "Root Canal Therapy Through Faith Healing." This may be even better than last year's great hit, "Two and One-Half Minute Root Canals Without Using Your Fingers."

Another instant classic could be "Rinsing with Borscht for Total Periodontal Therapy."

Not only would this remove periodontal pockets—but it acts as a great disclosing solution. You must make sure that the beet content is minimal and that the boiled potato is omitted.

Once you find the word or acronym which suits you, and get a lovely new technique, follow up by going to:

III. Literature and Flyers

This is what you know as junk mail and this is how to net the fish. Your mailing piece must be professionally prepared and costly so as not to be discarded before being assiduously perused.

Never use words like "assiduously perused" in your mailings—substitute "read." You have to hit them hard and fast, because six other mailings on great courses have also been delivered that day.

Use a professional advertiser, and get a great photo of yourself taken 10 or 15 years ago when you had hair. Write up a marvelous curriculum vitae (don't lie—embellish).

*Reprinted with permission from *Dental Management*, (Aug): 26–27, 1984.

IV. Course Location

Where the course is held is another integral part of your success story.

Use a hospital or dental school if possible. An amphitheater is great if one is available. If either of these are not available, make sure it's in a big city, or at least a place that doesn't have a funny sounding name like Piscataway, Walla-Walla, Succasunna, or Secaucas.

A fancy location will attract higher types.

V. Attire

First of all, you must look successful, but if you really are successful it doesn't matter how you dress. You can wear a turtleneck sweater, designer jeans and open-toed sandals or a shirt open to the waist displaying chest hair and gold (not silver) chains with religious medallions or symbols.

But if this is your first big chance on the circuit, you must appear understated and dress in the post-collegiate manner: a dark suit, buttondown shirt, striped tie, shined shoes. No silk handkerchief in the breast pocket—it is a sign of affectation.

Polyester leisure suits are out. You can overlook this last dictum if you are addressing a group in Miami, Fla., or Sun City, Ariz.

VI. Menu

This area is of great consequence. You must provide not only a luncheon, but coffee breaks featuring coffee, tea, and Danish pastries (or sweet rolls as they are called in the hinterlands).

The Danish selection should be eclectic: prune, cinnamon, cheese.

For the luncheon—no chicken or bland roast beef. This is the fare for every dental meeting ever held. Try avocado salads, nouvelle cuisine and the like. The meal should not be heavy—this will induce drowsiness and dyspepsia.

VII. Jokes

A little levity never hurt an all-day seminar. The jokes should be short, and even if they are slightly off-color, that's all right. Try to avoid ethnic jokes because someone's sensibilities may be bruised.

The best places to introduce your bon-mots are at the introduction, right after both coffee breaks and after lunch.

Good sources of jokes are bartenders, late-night TV, Joe Miller's Joke Book and funny friends.

If you have followed the logical steps outlined here—you can join the ranks of those dentists who have become household names. As always, the first step is the most difficult, but the rewards will be astounding.

Just imagine: 200 people attending a full-day seminar at $500 each person add up to a gross of $100,000 for the speaker. If you subtract the cost of the lecture room and the lunch, coffee and pastries, you still have a net of $98,432.78.

If you work six days a year—this will far exceed the half million dollar total. It will also allow you ample time to travel, play golf, pursue your hobbies, and even practice some dentistry.

If you have found this article to be of value—please send $500 to the author.

DENTAL INVENTIONS FOR FUN AND PROFIT*

Maurice J. Teitelbaum, D.D.S.

When a pastime becomes profitable, it's a complete joy. But this doctor's diversion didn't quite make it.

When a hobby becomes profitable, it is more than a pleasant diversion; it is a complete joy. So, with this in mind, I got to work with my Gilbert chemical set. After a few months I came up with a new revolutionary type of dentifrice.

It was great fun and now I was ready to put my toothpaste on the market and watch the money roll in. But things weren't quite that simple. The following correspondence will give you an idea of what finally happened:

Dear Dr. Teitelbaum:

It's always nice to receive a letter from one of my former chemistry students at the dental college. Enjoyed reading about your experiments on a new toothpaste. However, a dentifrice that just cleans teeth is hardly new and innovative and, frankly, is quite impractical in today's competitive market.

Since you are apparently interested in pursuing this idea and don't mind the hard work, I have a suggestion. Why not develop a toothpaste that is penicillinated, oxygenated, ammoniated, chlorophylled, bicarbonated, and fluoridated. It should also be homogenized, pasteurized and vitaminized. If you can see your way to incorporating the antihistamines, it would be a truly all-purpose toothpaste. Good luck.
                                          Professor Ossie Moses

Dear Dr. Teitelbaum:

Received your sample of the vitaminized all-purpose toothpaste. The flavor and odor are uniquely different; that is good. But the color is too commonplace; that is bad. If you can produce it in an original color we shall give it some consideration.
                                          Astigmatic Pharmaceuticals

Dear Dr. Teitelbaum:

Sorry, but I received seven ties last Christmas with the identical color.
                                          Astigmatic Pharmaceuticals

Dear Dr. Teitelbaum:

Thanks for sending us a sample of your all-purpose toothpaste. We like the color very much. In fact, we've adopted it for our company's banner, which is displayed Friday evenings at the Sunshine Bowling Alley during league competition. But the taste and the odor, ugh!
                                          Gourmet Pharmaceutical Company

Dear Dr. Teitelbaum:

We at the Homegrown Drug Company are definitely interested in your new toothpaste. Unfortunately, we have no facilities for its manufacture at this time. We have three warehouses filled with stale bread in preparation for our penicillin mold, and the philodendrons we use for making chlorophyll have started pushing up through the basement of our office building and threaten to invade the accounting department.
                                          Homegrown Drug Company

Dear Dr. Teitelbaum:

We regret having to return your sample. It is totally lacking in feminine appeal.
                                          Milady's Cosmetic Products

*Reprinted with permission from *Dental Management*, (Mar): 42–44, 1976.

Dear Dr. Teitelbaum:

So sorry, old chap. We detect a decidedly effeminate quality about your dentifrice. Actually, our clientele would never go for it.

British Esquire Products

Dear Sir:

We are very pleased with your new all-purpose toothpaste. There is just one small suggestion we should like to make. If you can design the tube so that the paste can be squeezed out in the shape of a cowboy on horseback we are prepared to place our order for 3,000,000 tubes.

Kiddy Products, Inc.

Dear Dr. Teitelbaum:

We are returning your sample dentifrice in a carton of recycled paper. We make our own all-purpose toothpaste which in addition to your stated ingredients contains rose hips, alfalfa, papaya, wheat germ, garlic oil, safflower oil, brewer's yeast, lecithin, bone meal, desiccated liver, sunflower seed extract, and raw peanut butter.

We haven't been able to market our product as yet because the smallest size tube into which we can fit our ingredients is 14½ inches long. This may seem a bit impractical, but we will not compromise when it is a matter of health.

Draw K. Cab Health Products
(Remember: Draw K Cab spelled
backwards is "Backward")

Dear Dr. Teitelbaum:

Congratulations! Your new toothpaste is the finest I have ever used. Mr. Hopkins and Mr. Worthmore, our second and third vice-presidents agree, and think it will revolutionize the dentifrice industry. Mr. Malone, our public relations man, is so excited about getting the advertising campaign rolling that he started looking up the telephone number of the *Reader's Digest*. Unfortunately, Mr. Jennings doesn't like it.

Leonard Lemonn, 1st Vice Pres.
Jennings Drug Company

Dear Dr. Teitelbaum:

Impossible for us to consider your product. Yesterday, bankruptcy proceedings were started against us. At present are only interested in sedatives.

Vanishing Cream Products, Inc.

Dear Dr. Teitelbaum:

Enclosed is $20 for your paste formula. We may be able to use it in our new skin cream.

Acne and Blemish, Inc.

Dear Dr. Teitelbaum:

We are in receipt of our check which you returned. Can make it $37.50 if you are interested.

Acne and Blemish, Inc.

Dear Maurice:

Uncle Harry and the children and I are fine. Thanks for the box full of toothpaste. Your uncle says that it isn't bad and he uses it. But he doesn't like the taste and says it smells like something that should be used under the arms. The children don't like it because they say it comes out of the tube like a snake instead of a cowboy on a horse. But they don't brush their teeth anyway. Please don't feel badly, I like the toothpaste very much. Please send more.

Aunt Hilda

THE SAGA OF DANNY DENTIST— ENTREPRENEUR *

Bernard P. Tillis, D.D.S.

Dr. Tilles was editor of the New York State Dental Journal *from 1972 until 1994.—Ed.*

You remember Danny Dentist
List' ye what his sad lament is
Saved his money, was most thrifty
Hoped that he'd retire at fifty.

He put his dough like any Moe into the bank
And stored the modest few percent with ne'er a
gripe
Until one night a colleague bright cried he was rank
To let such assets fallow lie when money making
schemes were ripe.

Danny mused, "I'm also ran'
Unless I find a better plan
If I'm to prosper when I'm older
My investments should be bolder."

He found a guy who wasn't shy with reputation
very shrewd
Who knew, 'twas said, his way around the stocks
on Wall Street
And Danny quaffed the glistening draught this fellow brewed
Paid cash he'd sweated out on aching feet.

Consolidated Sewer Pipe
Which had been the bullish type
Crashed the day that Danny owned it
Poorer Danny long atoned it.

A poorer even wiser man, Danny sought another
plan
To make his pile he would invest in some substantive real estate
For property would safer be, bethought himself our
clever Dan
He'd purchase land for which demand would rise
at some belated date.

Danny's land ne'er earned a cent
By sale or barter or by rent
Spared it was of brick or mortar
It idly lay there 'neath the water.

Growing older, he grew bolder, Danny sought to
make a killing
So when Willie Crackpot one day brought around
his new invention
Making toothpaste out of corned beef, he found
Danny eager, willing
To invest additional moneys, earn himself an old
age pension.

Corned beef toothpaste wouldn't sell
For while people loved the smell
They soon foreswore, would not abide it
Feared loss of teeth when they applied it.

Danny tried, his wits applied for many trying dental years
To accumulate that nest egg towards the day when
he'd go fishing
But savings earned by blood and sweat and even
tears
Wouldn't grow by wise investment, they simply always turned up missing.

Growing old is Danny dentist
List' ye what his sad lament is
"On a killing don't be bent
Be satisfied with 3 percent."

*Reprinted with permission from the *New York State Dental Jour-
nal,* (Jun/Jul):68, 1992.

SUNRISE, SUNSET*

Stewart Whitmarsh, D.D.S.

It seems an appropriate ending for this section—the writer announces his resignation as editor of the CDA Journal *and shares a few of his reasons.—Ed.*

My grandfather was a proper dentist. He was adjusting dentures for fifth-generation patients and napping between appointments when he finally retired at age 86. He lasted well into his 90s, well past my other ancestors, living proof that dentists have longer lifespans than horse thieves.

Taking a cue from my grandfather, I said many times in the last few years, "I'm far too young to retire. I enjoy dentistry. I'll just have a nice, quiet coronary over some poor devil in the chair and cause a commotion on my way out."

However, it's been 35 years of practice in Colorado, almost to the hour. One of the few friends I have left after being Editor of the *Journal* for four years, said, "Face it, you've joined the ranks of Geezerhood."

As I look back, I should have recognized the signs:

- I'm on my fifth dog and this one is ready to drop dead.

- I paid more for my 1995 car than my 1960 house.
- The kid dressed in the new airplane suit, greeting me respectfully at the door of the plane, turns out to be the pilot.
- For health's sake, I have become addicted to nutrition-rich foods, much of which tastes like kelp.
- Lately my physician has developed a keen interest in examining certain bodily parts which are too embarrassing to mention.
- Recently, when I walked into the Social Security office to get my share before the system crashes, a paraphrase of Pogo came to mind: "I have seen the geezers and the geezers is me."

Consequently I am retiring and have relinquished the Editorship of the *Journal* with great reluctance. By the time this issue is published, my wife and I will have moved to Florida, the land of alligators and mothers-in-law. . . .

*Reprinted with permission from the *Journal of the Colorado Dental Association*, 74(2):8–9, 1995.

TALES OF DENTAL EDUCATION

Dental school is the watershed event in a dentist's professional life. In four years, a raw student is transformed into an individual in whom the general public places enough trust to let the most neophytic dentist place a whirring, cutting instrument inches from the brain. Dentists have realized that education shouldn't end with the conferring of the DMD or DDS degree, and I don't know any practicing dentist who doesn't participate in some form of continuing education. This section contains pieces relating to all phases of dental education. Good luck with the "Bonus Question."

CONFESSION #14*

Dr. Richard Galeone

As I approach my fiftieth year, my demi-century, the final spike in the heart of my youth, it might be prudent to fess up to the sins of shame that soiled my soul and darkened my dental life. It seems so long ago that the rosy-fingered dawn of junior year descended upon us like an apocalypse and the instructors like Mongolian horsemen intent on ferreting out the weak and skewering the incompetent. Among this cadre of cavalrymen loomed tall and ominous one Rufus Quail, D.D.S., whose jerky prance and prominent Adam's apple soon gave rise to the pseudonym Rooster Man, a name that still causes an itching sensation in the nape of my neck.

It was a murky Monday morning in September when my Aunt Gessupina sat all atremble in the black and cream clinic chair, common sense having finally been overwhelmed by family loyalty. I had administered an anesthetic to the near vicinity of the mandibular nerve through taut muscle and was placing a #14 rubber dam clamp onto her lower left first molar. Gently, gently I removed the clamp holder from the clamp and let it hug the neck of her tooth. I took a piece of heavy rubber dam material, moistened the underside with a little lubricant, and started to maneuver it into position.

"Ooh, ooh," I heard from over my left shoulder. "Don't move. Leave everything exactly the way it is," said Rooster Man. "I'll be right back." And he ran off toward the black hole of his office.

Aunt Gessupina's goitered eyes rolled back in pre-epileptic alarm and, with what appeared to be bat's wings hanging from her mouth, was unable to ask me what irreversible mutilation I had performed on her anesthetized jaw.

Rooster Man returned with his camera and quietly announced to North America that he must take a picture to show his students how not to apply the rubber dam. I opened my mouth but was rendered mute, feeling it was fruitless to explain that the rubber dam was not on but rather was in the process of being put on. Instead, and to my everlasting shame, I prayed for a plague upon his progeny, a curse on the house of Rooster, and an infestation of locusts to be visited upon his children, yeah, and even to the seventh generation of the seventh generation.

Aunt Gesupina's eyes grew a map of varicose veins that looked like the Amazon Delta and a drop of sweat hung from the protrusion of her nose, a noble Roman prominence. Her look asked how she could have let herself fall into the hands of her brother's retarded son and spoke of the novena she would offer in thanksgiving for her safe liberation.

Flash. Flash. Flash. Rooster Man snapped from side to side adjusting the rubber dam so that there were points to the north, east, south and west, a black diamond on Aunt Gessupina's countenance. He advanced the film manually, and then, with a smug spin and not so much as a thank you, let alone an apology, returned Aunt Gessupina to my competent care.

I picked up the rubber dam frame and began to adjust the dam, downplaying to some extent the mortal wound inflicted upon the remnants of my ego. Curses, oaths and invective ricocheted crazily inside my head like goblins in a cave and my heart thumped in my ears like a sledge hammer on a drum. Rooster Man grew smaller in the lens of Aunt Gessupina's pince-nez.

As I continued to adjust the dam, Aunt Gessupina yawned in an attempt to reduce her nausea. With the stretching of her mouth the #14 rubber dam clamp shot out as if from a rifle and even registered the report of a little sonic boom. The sharp dagger-like wings of the clamp whistled through the air at eight hundred miles an hour and burrowed deep into the chaffed throbbing flesh on the back of Rooster Man's neck.

And behold, it is not by hard work and study alone that one advances through dental education, for in conspiracy with powers greater than ourselves we proceed toward state board examinations.

Bless me, Father, for I have sinned. I must confess that rather than admitting culpability for my obvious telepathic power, I groveled in feigned innocence under the accusing gaze of the Rooster Man's dilated eyes and only released myself to the pleasures of a sniggering giggle after he had been led away to have the #14, my favorite clamp, surgically removed from his neck.

*Reprinted with permission from the *Pennsylvania Dental Journal*, (Jan/Feb):56–57, 1993.

DENTISTRY'S DEMISE?*

Robert E. Horseman, D.D.S.

I don't want to alarm you unnecessarily, but there is an excellent chance that dentistry as we know it will come to an end sometime after the turn of the century, possibly in September. I learned about this impending disaster only recently when I received a letter from a Mrs. Finesia Otterstahter, a high school counselor from Port Landlock, Nebraska.

It seems Mrs. Otterstahter has learned of the closing of several dental schools and a general reduction in freshman class size, along with a diminishing applicants pool. She confesses that this state of affairs is largely her fault, hers and her fellow counselors. Since she had heard that I was the author of the dental version of the Hippocratic Oath and spokesman for the Abolishment of Spitoons and Zinc Chloride Based Mouthwashes, she felt she could come to me for absolution.

Well, not so fast there, Finesia. I remember the '70s too well, when you and your counselors managed to con thousands of otherwise normal kids into believing that their future lay in the profession of dentistry. These were kids who, until they learned from you what a sweet deal having a DDS behind their name was, would no more have thought of putting their hands in some stranger's mouth than they would of turning down the volume on their music. And as I recall, you were the one who talked me into taking two years of German and two years of Latin, failing to mention that everyone who spoke Latin was already dead and that the average German noun had 38 letters in it and gave you a sore throat if you tried to pronounce it. The only phrase I can remember after all these years is "Du bist verruckt in dem Kopf, mein Freund (you are crazy in the head, my friend)." Fortunately I never knew an actual German to say this to.

So anyway, by the time Mrs. Otterstahter and her cohorts, in concert with a government edict that dental schools receiving Federal aid must welcome all applying warm bodies, got done, the country was awash with dentists. Now Mrs. Otter-

stahter may claim she was a victim of demonic possession, with plenty of evidence to back her up, but the truth of the matter is that she and her ilk were largely responsible for the Great Dentist Glut of the Eighties.

When the counselors finally saw what they had wrought, the backlash set in. Now Mrs. Otterstahter admits that for the past couple of years she has discouraged even qualified applicants to dental school, suggesting they apply instead for positions in heavy metal rock bands or government service jobs where the only requirements are a double-digit IQ and the ability to tie your own shoes without detailed written instructions.

Applicant: I think I'd like to be a dentist.

Counselor (horrified): Have you considered coal mining? Your SAT scores and your aptitude tests indicate you would make a good assistant sheepshearer or shaving mug decorator.

Applicant: No, I think I'd like to try dentistry. I like to work with my hands and I like people.

Counselor: These are not people you're talking about. These are patients. They will spit on your fingers and harass you during Johnny Carson and Saturday afternoon football games. Eight years in college! You know what that means? Thousands of hours spent indoors when you could be surfing, and for what? To hear seventy thousand times a year, "I don't like dentists!" What are you, kid, some kind of masochist?

And so another promising youngster is lost to dentistry, gets into the entertainment business or professional mud wrestling, and first thing you know he's shopping on Rodeo Drive and leasing a Range Rover. Meanwhile, and this is the whole point of this article if I remember correctly, enrollment by qualified applicants (i.e., those with $20,000 tuition) drops until by September 2000, the freshman class could be held in a phone booth.

*Reprinted with permission from the *Journal of the California Dental Association*, 18(12):60–61, 1990.

What we've got to do is very carefully coach these high school counselors so they send us the kids with the right stuff, eliminating those with skulls having the density of bowling balls, encouraging those with the capacity to endure a 40-hour week of intense concentration in a 2 × 3 area, turning off those who can hardly wait to take out 2 full-page ads in the Yellow Pages and embracing the few who actually relished the idea of dissecting frogs and worms in zoology class.

We need to start worrying where the next generation or two of dentists is coming from, although I'm concerned about where my generation of dentists is going and when. Otherwise, I estimate that by September 2000, the pool will be empty and you and I will have to practice forever.

BONUS QUESTION

The Far Side*

Gary Larson

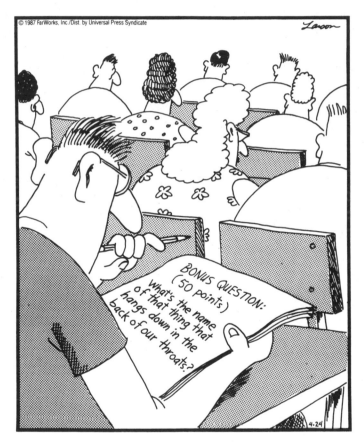

Final page of the Medical Boards

METERING DENTISTRY*

Robert E. Horsemen, D.D.S.

As I sink slowly into the twilight years of my practice (sort of on the order of a mastadon into the tar pits), I am pleased to discover that it is no longer necessary to maintain certain facades. If it turns out, as I suspect, that this is the only fringe benefit of aging, then it's worth it. Specifically, I refer to the charade I've had to support all these years of understanding the metric system of weights and measures.

I remember all too clearly that day many years ago, during my first week in dental school, when the instructor (played by Jack Palance) menaced the entire freshman class with these words: "All right, you people, lissenup! The whole profession of dentistry is based on one thing. You will learn this fact today and you will carry it with you for the rest of your life. It is the single most important criterion you will encounter every day, and if I ever catch any of you measuring **anything** with other than this, you will wish you were dead!" He paused, glaring into our innocent faces, then said, speaking in capitals for emphasis, words that seared our very souls, "I am speaking of THE MILLIMETER."

And he was right. The millimeter turned out to be somewhere between 1/16 and 1/32 of an inch, even though he would never admit it; and we did wish many times during those early weeks that we were, if not dead, at least far removed from his influence.

The millimeter was only the tip of the iceberg. It wasn't long before he was demanding we measure procedures in half millimeters and sometimes one-quarter millimeters. Now, a quarter of a millimeter is a single line of molecules and nobody in the class, including the instructor, had ever seen anything this microscopic. It was fortunate for us that our mentor had not heard of Murray Gell-Mann, who had discovered the quark while deciphering the deductions on his paycheck one day, or he would have had us putting 1/2 quark bevels on our inlay preps.

Instructors also loved the "micron." They used to tell us something was so many microns thick, but you could never confirm this by looking at it. To this day I feel it is simply too big a leap of faith to believe in microns. I'd sooner accept "no new taxes" and "cheerful refunds."

Well, time passed and eventually we came to accept, with prejudice, the millimeter. Those with a scientific turn of mind, who in their high school years ostentatiously carried around a really useless thing called a "slide rule," or as they smugly preferred to call it, a "slip-stick," embraced the millimeter readily. These were prototype dweebs and were beneath the contempt of the rest of the class.

The worst was yet to come. It evolved that 10 millimeters comprised a "centimeter" and 100 centimeters became a "meter" and so on until 1.609 kilometers became a mile. Can you imagine that? We already had a perfectly good mile that had been around for years and when someone exclaimed, "Boy, it'll go like 60!" everybody knew exactly what he meant. Try that with "95.54." Would you have walked 1.609 kilometers for a Camel—not now, of course, but back then? Don't be silly!

We can put the blame directly on Europe for fulminating all this confusion and then trying to foist it off on us under the guise of science. It started with the Visigoths, the Huns, the Celtics and the Forty-niners hoping to topple the English, who had built some swell castles and drawbridges with sensible inches, feet and yards even though they were having trouble with their money, which they insisted on measuring in quids, bobs, pence and ha'pennies. The European yahoos thought they could advance by using some things they made up called "grams," "kilograms," "liters" (which they couldn't even spell right, getting the "r" before the "e" as often as not), and to top it off they took 4,047 of their square meters and decided to call it "0.405 hectares." We finally figured out that what they meant was an acre, but

*Reprinted with permission from the *Journal of the California Dental Association*, 19(1):70, 1991.

that's about as close to a sense of humor as the Huns, etc., ever got. As a result they lived in caves and spent all their time plundering and pillaging and being unpleasant in groups of more than two because they hadn't even thought of the stall shower yet.

To be fair, we had some oddball measurements of our own which were probably brought over here by a moped dealer called "Amerigo" Vespucci because that was his name and who, because he came from Troy, had an ounce named after him. This irritated the French, who felt the ounce should be named after Avoir Dupois, inventor of the croissant, so they made their ounce heavier than the Italian ounce and today we in America can have a choice, and one that we wisely choose whenever we can remember which the hell is which.

There has been much agitation for many years to adopt the metric system in this country, but except for dental school, which, for lack of backbone, knuckled under immediately, and General Motors, which put an inner circle of kilometers-per-hour on its speedometers, which nobody ever looks at anyway, the efforts have played to an empty house.

Only one other profession is in more confusion than we are, and that's our friends the pharmacists. As a group, pharmacists are very disorganized, trying to be all things to all people. As a result, somebody has slipped the following into their frustrated lives: the "minum." It takes 60 minums to equal 1 fluidram, (ha, ha, no, I didn't make that up) and 2,400 to equal 1 "gill," so you can see how important **that** is. They've also got the "grain," the "scruple" and the "dram." Naturally, there is considerable doubt that these things actually exist. To test this, you might point a 9 mm pistol at a pharmacist's head some time and demand that he show you a scruple or two.

The point of all this is that for too many years we have been made slaves to a system that nobody understands nearly as well as a "smidgin," a "tad," a "pinch," and a "whole pile."

Keep the millimeter if you must, since you'd probably be lost without it now, even though a "teeny bit" is just as satisfactory for all intents and purposes, but please don't wait until life has passed you by to get out from under the yoke. And that goes for cubic milliliters, too.

DENTISTRY, GOLF AND SEX PROVE THAT PRACTICE DOES NOT MAKE PERFECT*

(and More "Official Rules" for Dentistry)
Randy Lang, D.D.S., D. Ortho.

The first "rules" that I can remember learning in dental school were G. V. Black's rules for cavity preparation. My classmates and I carefully memorized those rules along with hundreds of others that our professors and clinical instructors taught us.

But now, after many years in practice, I realize that the REAL "rules" for practicing dentistry are not taught to us in dental school, but instead must be learned in our offices after graduation.

I would like to share with you some of my favourite rules that I have learned—unfortunately, most of them the hard way.

- A mixing pad, if dropped while you're mixing cement, will always land cement side down. (This law was once tested in the Dental Clinic at the University of Toronto. Fifty students mixed cement on mixing pads and then tossed them up in the air. Forty-nine of the mixing pads landed cement side down on the floor. The fiftieth stuck to the cciling.)

- The chances of a new amalgam fracturing when the patient bites vary directly with the amount of time you spent carving it.

- Rules for office staff: 1) The dentist is always right. 2) When the dentist is wrong, refer to rule #1.

- Any gold crown or inlay, when dropped, will roll into the least accessible corner of the dental operatory and will not be found until the cement has hardened.

- Any sharp scaler or probe, when dropped, will always stab you in the leg on the way down.

- A sure way for you to get behind schedule is for your assistant to inform you that you're ahead.

- Office overhead rises to mcet income. It then passes it.

- The first 90% of a dental procedure takes 90% of the time and the last 10% takes the other 90%.

- More dental emcrgencies happen in your practice during the two weeks you are on vacation than during the 50 weeks you are there.

- All dental offices have a junk drawer. Anything wanted from the junk drawer will be found at the bottom. Once any item is removed from the junk drawer—no matter how large or small—the junk drawer will not close.

- The forecasting of dental manpower needs by the dental schools and government has made astrology look respectable.

- Any dental equipment or office machine that can go wrong, will go wrong, except when the repairman arrives, at which point it will magically, mysteriously (and temporarily) repair itself.

- If you take broken dental equipment apart to fix it enough times, you will eventually have enough pieces left over to build another one.

- Dental supplies always go on sale immediately after you have purchased them at the regular price.

- Your phone will not ring for the first 10 minutes of the day unless your receptionist is late, in which case it will ring continuously until she arrives.

- Good patients come and go. Bad ones accumulate.

- Patients' cheques are always delayed in the mail; bills arrive on time—or sooner.

- Eat a live toad first thing in the morning before going to the office, and nothing worse will happen to you for the rest of the day.

*Reprinted with permission from *Oral Health*, 85(9):3, 1995.

FAMOUS COURSES*

Richard B. Winters, D.D.S.

Each week via the mail we seem to be bombarded with a variety of brochures and flyers announcing continuing education courses, post-graduate courses, refresher courses, and special courses in all aspects, phases and specialties of dentistry.

The influx is endless and repetitious. After months of perusing the many different dental brochures, there is a pressing impulse to consign the unimpeded mass straight to the wastebasket, unread.

Every area of dentistry seems to have 2,832 experts presenting a course on the same subject, such as: "Wonderful World of Pin Restorations," "Wonder of Pins," "Pins and I," "What you Always Wanted to Know about Pins, etc," "Why Pins?" and "Why not Pins?"

To stem this confusion I have tried to gather a field of experts, each who have taken over 1,000 courses in the last twenty years, to compile and select the best courses in dentistry today.

The experts proudly present their compendium of Famous Courses:

Periodontics:

U_2: THE TURPIN TECHNIQUE: A COMPLETELY RATIONALIZED PERIODONTAL PROCEDURE.

Faculty: Ben Turpin, D.O.C., Charles Chase, D.D.S., Ben Blue, D.D.S., Edgar Kennedy, D.D.S., Leon Errol, D.M.D.

This one-day program will revolutionize periodontal therapy. It will demonstrate how an application of U_2 to the gingival tissues will cause shrinkage and tightening of all the tissues with successful elimination of periodontal defects and pockets with subsequent tightening of the teeth. Hours of periodontal therapy and surgery can now be eliminated entirely. A U_2 Kit[†] including a hydroscoper, acupuncture needles and 3 leeches will be sold at the demonstration-lecture.

(†*Due to the resemblance of U_2 to Preparation H, there may be some side effects that will be discussed at a subsequent lecture.*)

Tuition $500.00 Enrollment limited to 1,000. Lunch included.

Acupuncture:

ACUPUNCTURE FOR DENTISTS WHO ARE HAVING TROUBLE WITH LOCAL ANESTHESIA.

Faculty: Sidney Toler, D.D.S., Benson Fong, D.M.D., Mantan Moreland D.D.S., Key Luke, D.D.S., Fu-Manchu, D.O.C.D. (Doctor of Chinese Dentistry).

This course will discuss and demonstrate the ancient philosophy of acupuncture as a healing art and modality. It will treat the medical/legal aspects of acupuncture and its application as a tool of the dentist and a part of his everyday armamentarium.

It will be shown on charts and live models how the insertion and twirling of 75 strategically placed needles in the human body can produce the same effect as one local injection placed in the oral cavity.

Tuition $250.00 or 8 billion yen. Luncheon included: Mandarin or Cantonese (make choice on application). Enrollment: 250.

Practice Administration; Seminar Workshop Courses:

HUMAN RELATIONSHIPS SKILL AND TOUCH LAB FOR THE DENTIST AND AUXILIARY PERSONNEL.

Faculty: Harry Reems, D.D.S., Georgina Spelvin, D.A., Speed Vogel, D.D.S., Monte Blue, D.D.S., Arlana Blue, D.D.S. (husband and wife team).

The dynamics of the interpersonal relationships of the dental office health team will be examined as the basis of successful practice administration. Problem

*Reprinted with permission from the *Journal of the New Jersey Dental Association*, (Winter):16–17, 46, 1976.

areas "touched on" will include: role playing, problem solving, fooling around, conflict management skills, office tasks, costumes, sado-masochistic outlets, and group involvement. Office personnel and wives are encouraged to attend. Informal clothes are in order.

Tuition $100.00 per night. Dinner included. Enrollment limited to paired off groups. (300 people maximum).

Orthodontics:

THE PHILOSOPHY AND PRACTICE OF ORTHODONTICS WITH THE HOUDINI APPLIANCE.

Faculty: Harry Houdini, D.D.S., Melbourne Christopher, D.D.S., Milton Blackstone, D.M.D., I. Duninger, D.D.S.

Indications and therapeutic possibilities of the treatment with Houdini appliances of the various classes of malocclusion will be discussed with illustrated slides, films and X-ray demonstrations.

The practicality of the Houdini Technique will enable the practitioner to do away with extractions, banding of teeth and wiring. The principles involved will be concerned with the real and illusory manifestations of the appliance (which resembles a football helmet) in that the appliance will force the patients facial configurations and musculature to conform to the alignment of the dentition. Therefore, in a typical class II or class III malocclusion, the integral parts of the head and face will be rearranged.

This course is open to practicing orthodontists only.

Tuition $1,000.00. Enrollment limited to 25. Snack included. Time: 9:00 a.m.–9:15 a.m.

Endodontics:

PARTICIPATION COURSE IN 4-DIMENSIONAL FILLINGS OF ROOT CANALS—WITH LUKEWARM TO TEPID GUTTA PERCHA.

Faculty: Ambrose Schindler, D.D.S., Natty Bumpo, D.D.S., Beppo Schmidt, D.D.S., Elwood P. Dowd, D.D.S.

This course offers intensive clinical practice in this sensational technique which is 100% successful (as were the silver point, cold percha, and hot gutta percha techniques).

The participants will clean, shape, and fully prepare the canals for a four-dimensional type of filling and then obturate the canals on command. Note: This course is only available to participants in the three dimensional and semi-advanced courses that were previously given.

Tuition $250.00. Enrollment 12. Bring your own lunch.

Preventive Dentistry:

HOW TO PREVENT DENTISTRY ENTIRELY.
Faculty: Fred C. Dobbs, D.D.S., Wolf J. Flywheel, D.D.S., Hugo Z. Hackenbusch, D.D.S.

This course is given in conjunction with the National Dental Health Service where our fellow dentists and researchers are striving valiantly to eliminate all dental problems and ultimately dentistry itself. It is made possible by a grant from the Candy Makers of America.

The course is designed for the general dentist and his prevention therapist. Topics touched on will be: plaque control, nutrition, fluoride treatments, patient motivation and counseling.

The major breakthrough at the Institute has been the use of sealants which will be used to cover the entire dentition at the initial eruption of the deciduous teeth and then again as the adult dentition erupts.

There will be an auxillary course given in the retraining of dentists for other allied fields once dentistry is completely eliminated.*

*(*There will be a follow-up course on the buying and selling of apples including the different classifications such as: MacIntosh, Delicious, Winesap, Rome, etc.)*

Tuition: Free (First 500 applicants accepted). Bring your own lunch.

Practice Management:

HOW TO NET $100,000.00 A YEAR IN DENTISTRY WORKING 8 HOURS PER WEEK:
Faculty: Barnett Brodie, D.D.S., Isaac Gellis, D.D.S., Warner Baxter, D.M.D., Harlan Sanders, D.D.S.

The objective of this course is to inspire you to improve your practice by going from the dental treatment room out into the world of the lecture circuit.

Included in the curriculum will be:

(1) demonstrations on the construction of graphs and charts.

(2) visual aids.

(3) modalities of dress for lecturing (including color coordination).

(4) the correct etiquette for eating chicken, mashed potatoes, and green peas.

(5) the proper use of a slide projector and a pointer (use of a clicker is optional).

(6) choosing of titles for the lecture:

    (a) why you shouldn't use—"What you always wanted to know, etc."

    (b) why you shouldn't use such key words as "modality."

(7) choosing of proper environment for presentation (Howard Johnson vs. Holiday Inn).

Tuition: $500.00 Enrollment limited to 750. Lunch: Chicken, mashed potatoes and green peas.

THE THREE STOOGES*

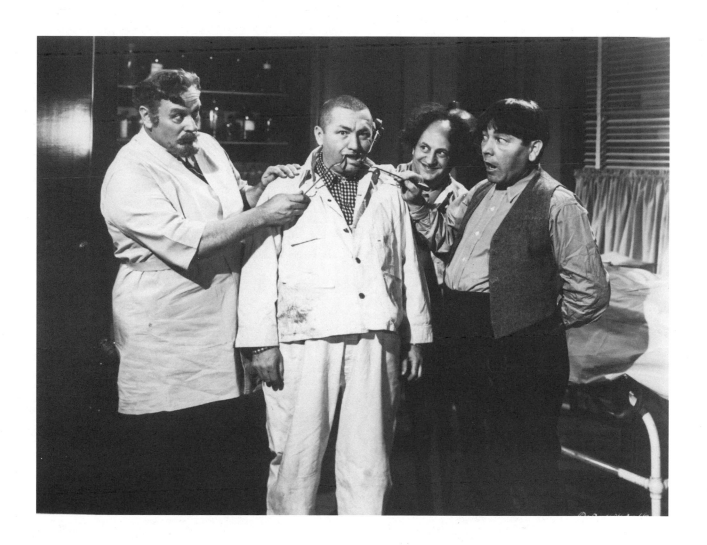

*Unknown short, approx. 1943. *With permission of Photofest,*
New York.

DISEASE, PATHOLOGY, AND RESEARCH

(And Other Things in Journals)

If all the papers published in dental journals in a single year were piled up, their height would exceed the total length of 1,469 periodontal probes laid end to end. While it is likely that most of these articles contribute in some way to the practice of dentistry or our understanding of disease, some contribute more than others. Some probably contribute only to the length of the author's curriculum vitae—or to our unread paper pile. Scientific method is sacrosanct, but it can still be fun to bend the rules.

MINIMUM INSTRUMENTATION FOR CONSERVATIVE OPERATIVE PROCEDURES*

Wilmer B. Eames, D.D.S.

When Black (1908) described the proximo-occlusal cavity preparation, instruments and philosophies of tooth reduction were such that gross cutting of the occlusal was advocated for strength and retention of the restoration.

A departure from this concept was described by Bronner (1930), who conceived and advocated a new conservative proximo-occlusal preparation. This preparation has been both acclaimed and criticized by many clinical investigators and clinicians.

Markley (1964) described a technique for minimizing the occlusal entry by using a No. 1/2 round bur with an ultraspeed handpiece—the premise being that the smooth shank cannot overcut the tooth. The preparation of the cavity is then completed with other burs.

An extension of this concept was proposed by Sturdevant (1964), who has initiated the manufacture of a No. 1/4 round bur (Kerr Mfg. Co., Romulus, MI 48174, USA). The use of this bur further points up the trend to greater conservation of tooth tissue in restorative dentistry.

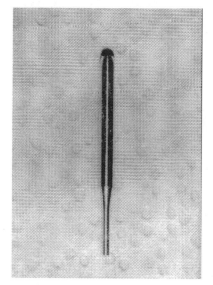

Figure 1. *The Aught series bur.*

Sequelae

It is here proposed that, to project the emphasis of conservative cutting to its utmost, the obvious instrument is the No. 0, or 00, bur (Montebank Dental Mfg. Co.). The No. 0 bur is indicated for the posterior teeth of adults and the No. 00 bur for posterior deciduous teeth. These burs will hereafter be referred to as the aught series bur (see figure).

Since the bur consists of a shank without the conventional head, it is suggested that the clinician use only the nondentated form, thus eliminating one more element of divective surface interphase.

The use of the aught series bur has been extended into many areas:

The most obvious operation for routine use is the preparation of congenitally missing teeth and deciduous teeth lost in playground altercations. It can further be used for the reduction of the fifth cusps of lower second molars and for the prophylactic odontotomy of the stained grooves of octogenarians who have not experienced previous dental caries.

A special use for the aught series bur is in removing clinically and radiographically nonevident caries—the bane of the enthusiasts of pit and fissure sealants. Its use has also been shown to eliminate the subsequent need for hand instrumentation.

Histologic studies have shown the No. 0 bur virtually to eliminate adverse response of the pulp during abusive cutting, with or without air or water coolants. The bur has, in fact, been found to be useful even when operated digitally. This has greatly enhanced the recent effort for more effective expanded utilization of auxiliary personnel.

Method of Testing

An effort was made to examine the effect of the eccentricity of this bur. Only production specimens, proffered during dental meetings, were tested.

*Reprinted with permission of the *Journal of the Colorado Dental Association*, 71(Apr):16–17, 1993.

DISEASE, PATHOLOGY, AND RESEARCH (AND OTHER THINGS IN JOURNALS)

Rotational speeds from 500 to 400,000 ± 4 rev/min with an air turbine handpiece were used as standards for all tests.

A tooth section to be used as a control was first photographed in profile and tru-casts recorded on a gross Blancetnuit dichrometer, as described by Day (1961).

To satisfy the conditions of the experiment, it must be assumed that the relationship between the SRO and the planing time is inversely exponential. In such a case, the SRO becomes a positive hyperbolic function, exceeding the 95% level of confidence.

The aught series bur eliminates the tendency for stress concentration in which the instrument may reach its frennic limit. Planning an infinite Cortwait will also increase the value of another variable, (CH)1, defined by the following equation:

$$*(CH)1 = \frac{C + an}{e^r} - y$$

Where:

(CH)1 = planing speed

C = cumulative surface froning

a = rate of decrease of planing speed with respect to surface poiuyt.

n = planning depth of bur when this value becomes constant.

e^r = parameter of infinity

y = a parameter of initial planing expediency.

[*Note: By the sheerest coincidence, this formula, when pronounced phonetically, gives credence to the dim but firmly held suspicion of incredulity.—Ed.*]

Interpretation of Data

It can be seen that as ultra speeds are approached, the eccentric quiescent phrases are absolved in the phase of oberlappen, as described by Wolfgang & others (1958). This phenomenon has been observed in almost total absentia, i.e., the fact that the nondentated characteristic of the aught series bur further obscures the true clinical impact of the Devinorm calculation.

The Pogrin Tider

The "Progrin Tider" is the key. It has never been used as a research tool before, but by all our scientific standards, is, and deserves the rank of entremanure.

A test analysis of variance was made of the degrees of probability. It was held that the consummate result clinically corroborates the view that the eccentricity as presently considered was tider or was, at the least, a pogrin tider.

It is not agreed that the "pogrin tider" can be adopted as a universal parametric descriptor for specification purposes at this time. While the evidence is weighty, the statistical method employed, a one-way AOV, is of questionable applicability. It would have been much more convincing had Barlett's test been used since this method has proven so valuable in prior bur research, at least with pear-shaped burs.

Discussion and Conclusion

The climate of this study could be unjustifiably altered by those who are inclined to carry it to an unrealistic parameter. It has been suggested that the bur could be useful in the range of 0.0 or 0.00, and even the exaggerated 0.00^0 has been considered. These are not thought to be practical and it is strongly felt that there is no support for this premise. The author is, however, currently investigating the obscure concept of the shankless aught series bur. The manufacture of this bur has become a problem. The clinician can well appreciate the complexities of producing such instruments, in that the ideal material for this bur has not been found. The production costs cannot be borne over a long-range program, because normal replacement due to wear and change of design is obviated. Initial cost of instruments may understandably be abnormally high, but would, of course, be compensated by a liberal annual cost-use ratio obsolescence, which could be introduced by any competent economic adviser.

We have every reason to expect that the aught

series bur may well provide the clinician with the ultimate in conservative operative nostrums—a real turkey.

The loss of a grant has obviated the exploration of new facets, but further studies need to be done.

References

Black, G. V. (1908) *Operative Dentistry.* Chicago: Medico-Dental Publ. Co.

Bronner, Finn J. (1930) Engineering principles applied to class 2 cavities. *Journal of Dental Research,* 10, 115–119.

Day, Thyme O. & Knight, Deado. (1961) Bisexual behavior of the beetle nut weevil. *Biodontographical Review,* 49, 161.

Markley, Miles R. (circa 1964) Personal communication. *Round Table Seminar—A Tax-deductible Consultant Conference.* Los Angeles: Pink Pussy Cat.

Sturdevant, Clifford. (circa 3/4:00 am) Personal communication. Chicago: Rush Street. *Ibid.*

Wolfgang, R. A., Messerschmitt, M. A. & Meisterbrau, Quorto. (1958) Preparation av klass II-kaviter. *Odontologica Levi Strauss,* 14, 92.

A MARGINAL STUDY OF THE RELATIONSHIP BETWEEN ORAL HYGIENE AND SYSTEMIC HEALTH*

Randall S. Asher, D.D.S., M.S.

Introduction

Every practitioner of dental science must constantly be vigilant in keeping the overall health of the patient as the ultimate goal of treatment. While multiple studies exist detailing physiologic effects of almost every aspect of dental care, very little has been done with regard to the relationship between oral hygiene procedures and systemic health.

It is the intent of this study to detail the type and magnitude of effects of oral hygiene procedures on the overall health of the individual. Data will be analyzed using multiple variant statistics and the Oberle 'U' introduced recently at the annual meeting of the International Association for Research Dentistry.[1] While the theory has existed for over 75 years, only recently has technology become available to properly use this powerful research tool.[2]

Materials and Methods

Data for this study were collected utilizing the Health Net[3] and Tooth Pix data bases.[4] The information parameters were defined by substantive need, as defined by the American Academy of Medical Terminology.[5] Only in this manner could the true potential of the data be completely maximized and properly applied to the epidemiologic situation as previously discussed.[6]

The data were separated at random into four different and distinct categories (see key):

    (1) Pressure intense oral hygiene devices, or OHDs (spot-specific);

    (2) Pressure intense oral hygiene devices (area-specific);

ORAL HYGIENE DEATHS 1979-1982

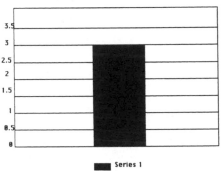

Figure 1. *Oral hygiene deaths 1979–1982.*

ORAL HYGIENE INJURIES 1979-1982

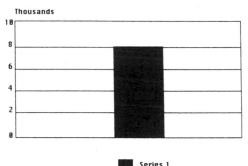

Figure 2. *Oral hygiene injuries 1979–1982.*

    (3) Low-pressure high-intensity liquid oral hygiene devices;

    (4) Multiple-tip manually-activated oral hygiene devices.

Results from each participant were tested against non-oral hygiene practicing, age and sex-matched controls from the school's main clinic.[7–10]

*Reprinted with permission from the *Journal of the Colorado Dental Association,* (Apr):31, 37, 1994.

The data were "scanned" into the Centerpiece data base using the For-Whom-the-Bell-Towles digital entry system. The results were the most efficient and error-free data entry in the history of our school.

Results

Analysis of the data showed some clear and highly significant trends. These trends are graphically represented in Figure 1s and 2. From this data it is clear that significant injury and even death has resulted from the use of spot-specific OHDs. It is obvious that the spot-specific OHDs result in some 8,000 injuries each year and have been responsible for at least three deaths. This is an incredible toll of death and injury in the pursuit of good oral hygiene.

The high-pressure, area-specific OHDs are mostly responsible for mutilation of gingival tissues and increased bacterial levels in blood. Unfortunately, it is not known if this increase in bacteria is significant.

While injuries suffered from area-specific devices were less severe, injuries from low-pressure high intensity liquid OHDs were significant in selected study subjects. It should be clearly noted that low-pressure/high-intensity OHDs contain large quantities of known dangerous elements such as alcohol and phenol. Each of these is associated with oral disease and long-term use, and are responsible for some 2,000 accidental poisonings each year.

Multiple-tip manual activated OHDs have been associated with increases in blood bacteria levels and are often found lodged in pharyngeal mucosa of toddlers. Interestingly enough, injuries sustained with the multiple-tip manually activated OHDs were restricted to the young.

Conclusion

From the data collected and analyzed using multiple variant regression analysis and the Oberle 'U,' a prudent health care provider can only ask the question: Is the price of good oral hygiene worth the cost in human suffering and death? Should these products be removed from the market and a campaign mounted to inform the public, in much the same manner as amalgam?

OHD Devices Key

(1) Toothpicks
(2) Floss
(3) Mouthwash
(4) Toothbrush

References

1. Leone E: Use of the Oberle 'U' in statistical analysis for health care. International Association for Research Dentistry, Annual Session, Zino poa Tibet, 1960–1970 IBID 1992 to present.

2. Dunn B: Manipulating the Oberle 'U' in the No Windows fluorescent light environment. *Journal of the Technowhiz* 2:24–36; 1993.

3. Health Net is a registered subsidiary and trademark of the Social Safety Net, a for-profit of the American Society for Deficit Spending (ASDS), Washington D.C.

4. *Tooth Pix*—a service of the National Association for Profit from Scrap and Kindling (NAPSAK).

5. Proceedings of the American Academy of Medical Terminology, May 5, 1994. Philadelphia, Pennsylvania.

6. Whitmarsh S: *Hitchhiking on the Information Super-Highway: A Tourist's Guide*. Denver, Full Court Press, 1993.

7. Spence P. The *toothpick* will get the job done. *Journal of OHD* (I)70–25–285. (II) Yosemite (So). 1993.

8. Kittleman W: Is *dental floss* the answer?" USSR *Journal of Mucosal Irritation and Oral Oncology* 45:36, 1994.

9. Steinhauer P: How much is enough alcohol in *mouthwash?* N Vietnam Journal of Mucosal Irritation and Oral Oncology 45:36, 1994.

10. *How to Make the Simplest Incident Exceptionally Complex—the Tooth Brush Incident: An Employee's Guide.* Department of Regulatory Agencies, Division of Ambiguity and Risk Management, Congressional Press, Washington, D.C.

CONTINUOUS FORCE INDUCED MEDIAL MOVEMENT OF THE EXTERNAL AUDITORY MEATUS AND AURICLE*

Laurence I. Barsh, D.M.D.

OSHA-mandated use of face masks in dental offices has initiated concern by the major manufacturers of these masks over the long-term use of elastic band ear loop retainers and their effect on the position of the auricle and the external auditory meatus itself. The amount of the elasticity necessary to retain the mask must be balanced against the potential "orthodontic" movement of the auricle and external auditory meatus caused by the continuous pressure exerted by the elastics when the mask is stabilized by the over-the-bridge-of-the-nose wire that is used to prevent eyeglass fogging.

This study was undertaken to determine whether or not movement occurs. Over the 36-month period of this study, the auricle and external auditory meatus was repositioned an average of 1.15 mm when elastic ear loop masks were worn 5 days per week for two 4-hour work periods separated by a 1 hour noontime removal of the mask.

Because of the public's increasing concern over the safety of dental visits and demand for employee protection, both the Centers for Disease Control (CDC) and the Occupational Safety and Health Administration (OSHA) have recommended that face masks be used for all dental procedures.[1] Because these masks must be removed and replaced frequently throughout the day in dental offices, the conventional surgical tie method of retaining these masks has been largely replaced by the more convenient elastic ear loop retaining device.

At a meeting of the Dental Manufacturers of America (DMA) in January 1989, concern was expressed over the potential effect of the "orthodontic" force of the elastic band retaining devices when the mask was stabilized by the over-the-bridge-of-the-nose wire that is used to prevent eyeglass fogging. This study was undertaken in May 1989 to determine whether or not movement of the auricle and external auditory meatus could occur induced by continual wearing of the elastic ear loop retaining device.

Materials and Methods

Thirty-eight dentists, ranging in age from 28 to 62, were divided into two groups. Nineteen dentists (7

of whom were female, 12 were male) agreed to wear ear loop retained masks for a period of 36 months. Masks were to be worn for two 4-hour periods daily over a five-day week for a total of 40 hours per week.

If the work week extended over 40 hours, the subjects wore to switch mask type to the surgical tie type mask. The control group of 19 dentists (5 female, 14 male) wore surgical tie type masks for the same period of time and were used as a control group and to measure the accuracy of the measurement techniques. Neither group was to take longer than four weeks vacation per year, and no vacation period could extend for longer than eight consecutive days. Subjects were asked not to consciously alter their weight (dieting was not allowed) during the course of the experiment.

A tiny spot was tattooed, with black ink, on the tragus of the ear of each subject as well as on the alar of the nose and at the outer canthus of the eye on the right side (Figure 1). Because the relative difference in position of each tattoo was to be measured, the exact positioning of the tattoo from subject to subject was unnecessary. Using the relative difference between points rather than exact measurements standardized the measurement between subjects with different facial sizes.

A line was drawn from the tattoo on the tragus of

*Reprinted with permission from the *Journal of the Massachusetts Dental Society*, 41(4):169–171, 1992.

DISEASE, PATHOLOGY, AND RESEARCH (AND OTHER THINGS IN JOURNALS)

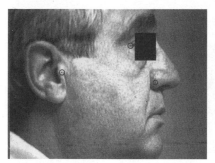

Figure 1. *Subject #12 with tattoo marks (indicated within black circles) on the tragus of the ear, alar of the nose, and outer canthus of the eye.*

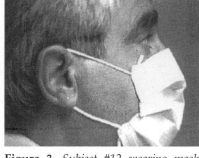

Figure 3. *Subject #12 wearing mask with ear loop retaining device used in the experiment. This brand was worn during the extent of the experiment.*

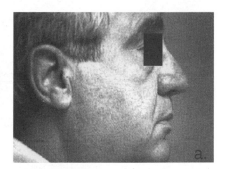

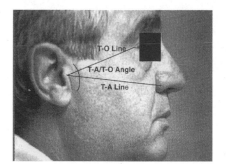

Figure 2. *Subject #12. T-O and T-A lines have been labelled. The T-A/T-O angle is indicated.*

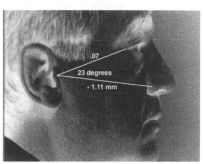

Figure 4. *Subject #12 at end of experiment. The T-O line length had increased .07 mm. The T-A line had been decreased in length by 1.11 mm. The T-A/T-O angle increased from 16 degrees at the start to 23 degrees at the completion of the experiment. Illustration shows negative image upon which measurements were made.*

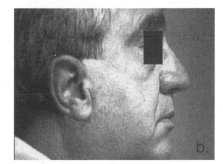

Figure 5. *Subject #12 at the start (a) and completion (b) of the three-year experimental period. Although results were not this dramatic on all patients, please note the downward and forward movement of the auricle and external auditory meatus.*

the ear to the tattoo on the alar of the nose. This is labelled the T-A line. Another line was drawn from the tattoo on the tragus of the ear to the tattoo at the outer canthus of the eye. This is labeled the T-O line. The T-A/T-O angle was also measured (Figure 2).

Two brands of readily available masks were utilized (Figure 3). The brands of mask were not changed throughout the course of the experiment. No attempt was made to standardize the elasticity of the ear loops during the course of the experiment because variation in quality control would occur in normal usage.

The subjects agreed to come to the investigator's office at 6-month intervals. To standardize the measurement technique and eliminate variables caused by three-dimensional measurement, measurements were made on standardized photographs of the subject. The subject's head was retained by ear plugs in

a conventional head retainer used for cephlometric measurement which was secured to the ceiling in the investigator's office.

An 8 × 10 studio view camera which produced a life-sized negative was mounted on a tripod secured to the floor. A 240-mm lens was used to photograph the subject to eliminate photographic distortion caused by a shorter focal length lens. The focus of the lens was fixed by drilling a small hole through the focusing ring and retaining the position of the focusing ring with a Hex head Bråne-mark implant screw.

All adjustable stages of the studio camera were fixed in a similar manner. Distance from subject to camera was 6.8 feet. Kodak Plus-X 8 × 10 fine-grain, black and white sheet film was used and processed in Dektol with controlled time and tem-

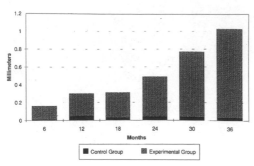

Figure 6. *Measurements along the T-A line in millimeter difference between original measurement and time dated measurement.*

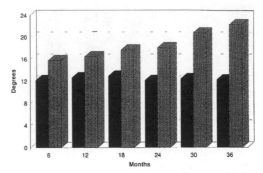

Figure 7. *Increasing obtuseness of angle between T-O and T-A line.*

perature. The black tattoo spot at each of the three locations appeared as a minute, punctate white spot on the negative. Measurements were made on the negative itself to eliminate shrinkage from drying contact prints on paper.

Measurements were made in both the experimental and control groups of the imaginary line from the tragus of the ear to the alar of the nose, from the tragus of the ear to the outer canthus of the eye, and of the angle between these lines in an attempt to determine the amount and direction of movement that occurred when continuous force was applied by elastic ear loop retainers (Figure 4).

Results

Over the 36-month experimental period, movement of the auricle and external auditory meatus occurred under the continuous loading applied with elastic ear loop retainers and proven by the loss of approximately 1.15 mm in the distance between the spot tattooed on the tragus of the ear and the alar of the nose in the experimental subjects (T-A line). While there was not statistical difference in the actual measurement made from the tragus of the ear to the outer canthus of the eye (T-O line), the angle between the T-O line and the T-A line became more obtuse indicating a downward and forward movement of the auricle and external auditory meatus (Figures 5–7).

Slight variations in measurements did occur in the control group, but these were within standard deviation and were statistically invalid. The variation was attributed to minor error in experimental technique.

Conclusions

It is evident that more research must be done to determine the proper amount of loading that can be applied to the distal-most portion of the auricle by the elastic retaining loops of commercially available face masks. The data presented confirm that the auricle and external auditory meatus move in a downward and forward direction under the continuous loading produced by these elastic ear loops.

Manufacturers must analyze the amount of force applied and critically balance the amount necessary to retain the mask against the possibility of movement. Although not tested by the courts as yet, it will be interesting to determine whether OSHA considers movement of the auricle and external auditory meatus, admittedly a purely cosmetic alteration, as a potential workplace injury.

References

1. Munchausen BV: Concerning the relative ease of placement of fictitious articles in peer adjudicated journals. Bull Soc Health Involved Teachers 12(3)194–99.

2. Personal communication, L. I. Barsh, 1992.

THE TEETHING VIRUS*

Howard J. Bennett, M.D.
D. Spencer Brudno, M.D.

A prospective study was carried out on 500 teething infants which demonstrated that a new infectious agent, the human teething virus, is responsible for the febrile response that accompanies the eruption of deciduous teeth. Speculations are made concerning whether or not amoxicillin should be prescribed instead of Jack Daniel's to treat teething infants and their parents.

Introduction

Teething has been the subject of intense interest in the medical and nonmedical community for centuries.[1] Controversy has resulted not only over the signs and symptoms associated with teething but also over the tooth fairy's impact on the family.[2,3] But perhaps the greatest controversy of all is whether or not teething causes fever. Unfortunately all of the research in this area suffers from serious methodologic flaws. McCartney et al.[4] reported that teething was responsible for fever in 20% of infants with temperatures $\geq 40°C$. That study was carried out in an emergency room setting, however, and therefore is not applicable to all infants. In addition, the authors failed to quantitate the amount of drooling that residents had to contend with and whether or not this interfered with optimal observation of the patient. More recently, Shorts[5] examined 240 teething patients in a suburban practice and concluded that teething does not cause fever. His population included school-aged children as well as infants, however, and it is well known that older children will feign illness in order to get stickers and other rewards from the doctor's office.[6]

Early in 1982 one of us was doing histopathology research on the brain cells of hairless mice that had been subjected to 36 hours "on-call." Inadvertently a sample of saliva from a teething infant (via a soggy bagel) was put under the electron microscope. To our amazement this accident uncovered a new viral particle (HJ Bennett, unpublished revelation). This discovery led to the diversion of all previously acquired grant funds into the search for the mythical teething virus. In this report we present the results of a prospective study of teething infants and young children undertaken during the Washington, DC, teething outbreak of 1983 and 1984. We report our findings, which prove conclusively that the human teething virus (HT virus) is the hitherto elusive agent responsible for the fevers associated with teething.

Patients and Methods

The study included 500 infants who were followed prospectively from birth through 2½ years of age. The patients were selected from consecutive term births at our medical center. Primiparous women were interviewed by one of the authors sometime during the third trimester—usually on the way to the delivery room. The mothers-to-be were asked two questions regarding possible entry into the study: (1) If you have a baby, would you like to participate in a study of teething in infants? (2) Do you believe in Santa Claus? A positive response to either question made the infant eligible for the study.

A total of 506 mother/infant pairs were initially included in the study. The patients were matched for socioeconomic status, educational background and whether or not both parents watched "Dallas" on Friday nights. Two infants with natal teeth were subsequently excluded, though it is worth noting that in both cases the mother experienced a "warm uterine feeling" 2 weeks prior to delivery. An additional four babies dropped out of the study for unknown reasons. Their mothers reluctantly withdrew from the project as well.

Mothers were instructed to bring their baby to

*Reprinted with permission from the *Pediatric Infectious Disease Journal*, 5(4):399–401, 1986.

the clinic at the first sign of teething. During this visit vital signs were taken and the infant was examined for physical evidence of teething using the method described by Leech.[7] Briefly, this technique involves having the infant breastfeed for 5 minutes in the office. If the mother's cry exceeds 90 dB, the baby is teething. The threshold is adjusted to 120 dB in nonnursing mothers. Infants were seen regularly during the teething period, and parents kept a diary of relevant symptoms.

Saliva was obtained on the fourth and sixth teething days by adsorption onto teething rings impregnated with human embryonic lung and human embryonic kidney. The specimens were processed using a revolutionary technique that is currently under investigation by a rival laboratory and therefore is not available for publication. Additional saliva was obtained from the subjects' mothers and in between episodes of teething such that each patient served as his or her own control. Serum specimens were not obtained due to parental squeamishness. All subjects and specimens were handled in a triple blind fashion: patients did not know why they were in the study, technicians did not know what was being studied, and the authors didn't care but hoped to get published anyway.

Results

Basic Research

The HT virus is a uniquely shaped viral particle with a diameter of 140 nm. The envelope surrounds a helical nucleocapsid that is covered with spherical studs (Fig. 1). Though superficially resembling a slice of white bread, the HT virus is actually the

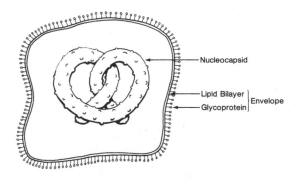

Figure 1. *Schematic representation of the human teething virus.*

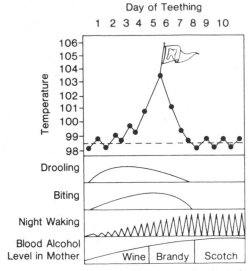

Figure 2. *Schematic diagram illustrating the clinical sequence of teething.*

first recognized member of a new family of RNA viruses to be named the Masticoviridae. Details of the virus' lifestyle and reproductive habits will be the subject of another report.[8]

Clinical Research

The 500 patients in our study experienced repeated bouts of teething during the first 2½ years of life. Teeth erupted at a rate of approximately 10 per year, which provided us with 5000 tooth-years of data. Eighty-four percent of patients became febrile during the teething process. The clinical course of these patients is shown in Figure 2. All patients recovered uneventfully from this developmental nuisance. Unfortunately, however, at least 15 divorces could be directly attributed to "irreconcilable differences" on how to manage a teething baby at 3 o'clock in the morning.

The HT virus was isolated by electron microscopy from well over 99% of febrile teething patients (Table 1). In fact there was only one febrile infant in whom the HT virus was not isolated, and the technician who handled that specimen admitted to misplacing the patient's teething ring and secretly testing his own saliva (J Cama, personal confession). The HT virus was not isolated from any of the nonfebrile teething patients, though it was seen in two samples taken from the mothers' group. In both cases, however, the mothers admitted to kissing their febrile babies just prior to submitting their own specimens for study.

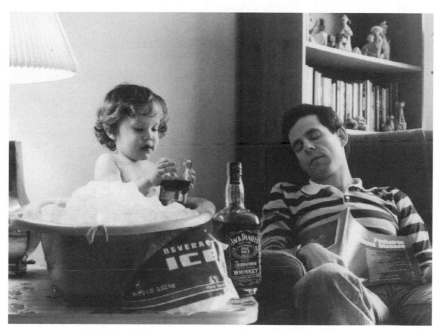

Figure 3. *The modern treatment of teething: an ice and alcohol bath.*

Table 1. Isolation of the human teething virus by electron microscopy in control and teething patients.

Group	No. of Samples Tested	No. Positive for HT Virus	% Positive for HT Virus
Mothers	500	2	<1
Nonteething infants	1000	0	0
Nonfebrile teething infants	800	0	0
Febrile teething infants	4200	4199	>99[a]

[a]$P<0.000001$ by Toddler's t test and the Fisher-Price test.

Discussion

Infants acquire their primary teeth by 30 months of age. Teething occurs off and on for 24 of these months—mostly on, according to parents. We have shown that 84% of infants develop fever when teething and that it is the HT virus which causes this fever. There appears to be little doubt, therefore, that parents have been right all along. Fortunately, however, teething phobia can now be approached intelligently instead of with the irrational treatments of the past (Fig. 3).

A few questions still remain, however, concerning the pathogenesis of the HT virus. We believe that primary infections with the virus occur early in life in the majority of children. These infections are probably subclinical most of the time but undoubtedly are also responsible for many of the "idiopathic" conditions of infancy, colic and difficult temperament, to name a few. Once the primary infection subsides, the virus becomes dormant within the alveolar ridge. Then, at future points in time, the aggressive movements of erupting teeth disturb the sleeping virus who retaliates by producing local and systemic effects. The pattern of transmission is not horizontal, as one might expect, but gravitational, this of course owing to the aerodynamics of drooling babies.

As a result of this study, we have revised the anticipatory guidance given at 6 months of age. Parents are encouraged to check for teething at the first sign of fever and to quickly begin their prophylactic Valium® if the baby's Leech test is positive. Finally we recommend that practitioners approach their 2 a.m. calls as a time to educate parents about the positive aspects of teething.[9] This advice will minimize the hoarding of left-over amoxicillin until such time as a vaccine is developed to rid mankind of this pesky little virus.

Acknowledgments

This work was supported completely by a grant from the makers of Orajel® and Goldstein's Bagel Shop. Special thanks to Judith Ratner, M.D., who somehow found the time to review our manuscript in between pelvic examinations in her adolescent clinic.

References

1. Radbill SX: Teething as a medical problem: Changing viewpoints through the centuries. Clin Pediatr 4:556–559, 1965.

2. Skinner BF: The tooth ransom: Are today's children holding out for too much money? J Pediatr Bribery 86: 314–316, 1980.

3. Westheimer R: Is 50¢ a tooth enough to get children to sleep in their own beds at night? J Parental Celibacy 69:123–128.

4. McCartney PL, Flintstone F, Rubble B, et al: Do teething infants need a CBC and blood culture? J Dubious Invest 59:463–468, 1977.

5. Shorts RH: Teething and fever: Another myth debunked. PMD Bull 21:459–463, 1982.

6. Munchausen BV: Factitious teething as a means to visit the pediatrician. Acta Idiotica Scand 70:212–213, 1978.

7. Leech LA: The clinical application of breastfeeding reflexes: "Let-down" means the milk is in, "Let Go!" means the teeth are coming. The Breast 36:24–34, 1982.

8. Bennett NJ, Brudno DS: The masticoviruses: Have we bitten off more than we can chew? Popular Virol, in press, 1986.

9. Weissman MI: Tootharche, menarche, and anarchy: Three developmental milestones of childhood and adolescence. Curr Prob Nightcall 12:1–7, 1983.

CASE HISTORY A LA MOOD*

Marc Tyler

Pick up any one of your scientific dental journals and read one of the case histories. A week later, try and remember what it was all about. It's a contra angle to a box of carding wax you can't. Why? Because it's dull reading. There's no style, no imagination. Read one case history of an impacted molar and you've read them all. But with a little imagination to create the proper atmosphere and mood, and with just a little bit of literary style, a case history would cling to your memory as tenaciously as an Ellery Queen murder mystery. For example, a case history a la mood might conceivably go something like this:

Patient: Mrs. Emily Newlywed.

Age: 29 years.

Present complaint: After hours of questioning, Emily, ashamed and in tears, decided to tell all. It was her husband's idea, she cried, the man she had married just two months ago.

"Your husband?" I asked. "But I don't understand."

"You see, doctor, he complains that . . . that . . ." Her voice choked up, she couldn't go on.

"Please, Mrs. Newlywed, try to control yourself. We want to help you, but we can't help if you won't cooperate with us. Come now, tell us everything, and it will be held in strictest confidence."

The patient braced herself, wiped her tear-stained face with a daintily embroidered Madeira handkerchief and began. It was her husband, she repeated, her husband had stopped making love to her. He had said that he couldn't go on with the marriage, for every time he tried to kiss her he suffered severe pain and laceration of his lip. A terrible situation, indeed, but unfortunately true! For even an untrained observer with the most casual glance couldn't help but notice the mass of fang-like upper anterior teeth that protruded a full three inches from the mouth of the unhappy woman.

Diagnosis: The secret was out at last, and Mrs. Newlywed was relieved of the burden that had weighed her down these past eight weeks. She tried to relax, but it was impossible. As hard as she tried, she could not bring her lips together. They had been strangers all her adult life, kept apart by the huge protruding maxillary teeth and they refused to come together even now.

There was but one solution, removal of the uppers, an alveolectomy and the insertion of an immediate partial denture. And in her heart, Emily Newlywed knew that she must make a choice. It was either her teeth or her husband! She weighed the decision carefully. Her teeth, she thought, had been part of her very being for 20 years—firm, steady and outstanding. And her husband, she had known him but a short time, yet it was with him that she had to build her future life. Finally, the hour of decision had arrived, and she decided that the teeth had to go!

Operative Procedure: The denture was prepared a few days earlier, and now it was time for the operation. Nervous and distraught, Emily seated herself in the chair. This was a great moment in her life. Had she made the right choice? Would her husband, John, love her after the operation, as he had before they were married? Was it really those mammoth teeth that had driven them apart or was it something else—or someone else!

Suddenly she was seized with panic as she thought of Helen, John's secretary. Helen had been separated from Bill, and she knew that Helen would stop at nothing to take John away from her. Emily wanted to get off the chair, and run out of the office, to run away from John and away from herself. Then she stopped struggling, her breathing became even and regular as the nitrous oxide dragged her down into the blackened, swirling whirlpool of the subconscious. The incision was made quickly, and the tissue was laid back exposing the alveolus. Cold steel was laid upon the coronal portion of each tooth as they were removed uneventfully. Then, with the rongeur and bone file, the dense buccal plate was clipped and trimmed.

*Reprinted with permission from *Tic*, (May):8, 15, 1985.

DISEASE, PATHOLOGY, AND RESEARCH (AND OTHER THINGS IN JOURNALS)

To Emily Newlywed, the humming noise became louder and louder as the hazy colors floating by took on the appearance of dancing figures. Her head was bursting with joyous laughter as a myriad of faces rushed past her. Then teeth showered down from the sky, and danced around her in a frenzy, gnashing at her as they dipped and turned. Now frightened and horrified, she tried to run away but her feet froze, and she felt herself sinking into the earth. The more she struggled to free herself, the firmer she became entrenched in the muddy clay. The noise grew louder and louder, and then she screamed. Formless people came rushing to her assistance. She could hear voices, at first jumbled and distant. Then she heard pleas to wake up, asking her how she felt and telling her it was all over. Then she smiled. She didn't know why, but she smiled. Slowly Emily opened her eyes. The smile was still on her face. As tears flooded her eyes, she noticed smiling faces before her. She started to cry quietly. Then her head cleared and she knew where she was, and that it was all over. There was a strange feeling in her mouth. She parted her parched lips and then closed them. They touched! At last she could bring her lips together! She wondered what she looked like, her mouth felt full. What would John think about her now? Was the operation a success?

For the concluding episode, read next week's *Journal* on the prognosis of this interesting case. In the meantime, tell your colleagues about it, they won't want to miss the exciting conclusion of this story, and the beginning of a new case history entitled, "How Green Was My Formen Ovale."

GOODBYE, CANKER SORES*

Donald F. Bowers, D.D.S.

What my mother called "canker sores," is now designated "MiRAS" or "MaRAS." According to a recent article in the *Journal of the American Dental Association* (JADA), you can call it MiRAS, if the sores are minor, or MaRAS, if they are major. Pretty simple, eh?

What I want to know is: What happened to canker sores? I asked that same question several years ago when the periodontists started to call the nasty little devils "recurrent aphthous ulcers."

A little later, the periodontal in-crowd began to refer to them as "RAU." I know a periodontist named Rau and, at first, I thought they had named a new disease after Charlie.

Periodontists tend to change the names of the diseases they treat from time to time. I think it gives them a sense of accomplishment and something new to talk about at meetings.

My grandfather lost his teeth because of pyorrhea. If he had lived a couple of generations later, he might have kept them because nobody has pyorrhea anymore. The disease has apparently been conquered. So has periodontosis. So has trench mouth. All of these have gone the way of trauma from occlusion . . . or was it occlusal trauma?

Now when I see a patient complaining about pain from a little ulcer (5 mm or less) surrounded by a distinct, raised and erythematous border, located in his or her labial vestibule, I can announce, "Well, it looks as though you have MiRAS."

"Oh, my gosh, I have MiRAS," the poor soul will say in a quavering voice. "Is it cancer? AIDS? I thought I just had a canker sore."

"Nobody has canker sores anymore," I'll say. "But not to worry. MiRAS is not serious. It could be worse. You could have MaRAS.

MaRAS won't kill you either but it lasts longer than MiRAS. And neither MiRAS nor MaRAS is nearly as painful as NUG."

"Praise the Lord," the patient will say after a sigh of relief. "I guess I'm plain lucky to just have MiRAS and not MaRAS or NUG."

"Boy, I'll say," I'll say. "But while I have you in the chair, I want to check you for CLIDE."

"CLIDE?" the patient will ask anxiously. "What's CLIDE?"

"CLIDE stands for carious lesion in dental enamel," I'll explain.

"Is that like tooth decay or cavities?" the patient will ask.

"Yes, it's like that," I'll proclaim proudly, "but we've conquered tooth decay. Nobody has cavities anymore, just CLIDE."

*Reprinted with permission from the *Ohio Dental Journal*, (Spring/Summer):3, 1991.

SAME MUSIC, DIFFERENT WORDS*

Edward Samson, F.D.S.

No sooner had someone discovered plaque in the dental vocabulary, than our scientific (and other) authors, delighted to have found a change of subject, set their typewriters working furiously; and dental journals were covered with more plaque than the nation's un-brushed teeth. And not surprisingly, since dentistry discovers too few stimulating novelties not to pounce avidly upon one when it makes a lucky appearance. Think only how long we have had to make do with fluoridation.

Expectedly, our American colleagues also jumped enthusiastically upon plaque, and with characteristic thoroughness, write about and discuss all its aspects and, of course, relate it to psychodontics, patient motivation, dentist/patient relationship, and all else that its new-found importance seems to deserve. Few of their journals fail to mention plaque control, plaque deposit, plaque-consciousness (of patients, not authors), and other manifestations of plaqueodontics.

One essay in the *Journal of the American Dental Association* particularly fascinated me. Most remarkable was not the two authors' evident delight in being able to extend plaque study, but their repetition of all those maxims we used, long ago, to apply to the simple exercise of toothbrushing. This instruction in oral hygiene, and the best way to teach it, I was taught and used in those distant days when dentists could find little to discuss but caries and 'pyorrhœa.' Now, it seems, the same things are being said about oral hygiene, except for debris, read dirt, and food deposit, read plaque.

Here in this essay, impressively titled 'Motivation—Key to Patient Success and Mechanical Plaque Control,' the authors tell us at the outset, 'Motivation of patients toward effective plaque removal requires the establishment of an effective dentist/patient relationship and proper instruction.' This I loosely interpret as meaning, 'Good teaching and good understanding between them is necessary.' And in case we miss the point, they quickly add, 'A positive re-lationship between the dentist and patient—good rapport—must exist to bring about any change in behaviour.' This is obviously most important since 'Motivation of persons who were previously lax about their oral hygiene necessitates a behavioural change,' which, I guess, means they must change their ways. And just to lend authority to their opinions, the authors quote the notable discovery of 'Korsch and co-workers' who 'showed that an important attribute of the pædiatrician, in establishing a positive relationship, was his communication skill.' This supports the authors' belief that 'In a positive dentist/patient relationship, the dentist is able to effectively communicate his instructions to the patient.' All this certainly makes the conditions for teaching patients abundantly clear.

So much emphasis on the way to tell people how they ought (dare I say it!) to clean their teeth. I feel, and with no disrespect to our authors, that Humpty Dumpty might add his conclusion to their treatise thus:

> *I said it to them, I said it plain,*
> *And I shall say it all again.*
> *I said it very loud and clear*
> *Just in case they might not hear,*
> *Though what I say is quite the same,*
> *At least it has another name.*

Possibly I am out of touch with contemporary dental thought, for I believed that, whether debris, dirt or plaque must be removed from teeth, the same method serves, even with the addition of the (new?) process Americans call 'flossing.' We are also presented with what, to some of my very young juniors, must be a novelty. 'For small children an effective reward often is a prize or award such as membership of a "clean-tooth club".' Do I remember Gibbs' 'Giant Decay' and the badges children wore to show they would take up their toothbrush to defend their 'ivory castles'? Let us,

*Reprinted with permission from the *British Dental Journal*, 143(1): 33–34, 1977.

then, have 'Giant Plaque,' and dental history will have come full circle. Moreover, however patients are encouraged or persuaded (that is, motivated) it is essential that 'the patient must be motivated to carry them (the instructions) through on a long-range basis' or, one might say, keep up the tooth-cleaning.

How fortunate for dental authors there are so many different ways of saying the same thing—variations on a theme. With the uneasy feeling that I have been here before I read of 'the uses of rubber dam,' or 'contamination of root canals,' or 'the expansion of dental amalgam,' or 'sugar intake and dental caries' and, of course, of 'effective communication.' And of every subject which, like the reader, should have been exhausted long ago. No wonder researchers are hard put to discover something new, and are driven to such esoteric matters as the 'Addition of various salts to cariogenic diets in rats.' May plaque long continue to inspire our authors, for there is nothing else in sight, unless it is time for an instant retake of—guess what!—caries, or an action replay of root canal filling (endodontics).

THE TMDEVIL'S TMDICTIONARY*

Robert W. Gear, D.D.S.

(With apologies to Ambrose Bierce and to the Random House College Dictionary.)

TMDabbler. 1) A patient who hates being left out of the latest disease fad and wants to try it out. 2) A dentist who hates being left out of the latest disease fad and wants to try it out.

TMDagger. *Syn:* Scalpel. Often used to destroy joints. Occasionally necessary.

TMDakoit. In India and Burma, a *dakoit* is a criminal who engages in robbery. The TMDakoit is a legalized version in this country. It mainly consists of dentists who charge too much for too little. Main victims are insurance companies and gullible patients.

TMDalliance. A trifling away of time; dawdling. The TM variant is used as a ploy to prolong treatment either because the schedule is slack, or because the treating TMDentist has no idea how to proceed.

TMDamage. 1) What adolescent girls do when they chew gum incessantly. 2) What yuppies and middle-aged women in unhappy marriages do when they clench their teeth. 3) What drinks do in Saturday night barroom brawls. 4) What some dentists and surgeons do who either don't know or don't care what they're doing to their patients.

TMDamages. Money collected by greedy attorneys and (occasionally) deserving patients from dentists and their insurance companies. The correlation between the dentists who are truly negligent and the dentists who lose the cases is only somewhat approximate.

TMDamsel. Gum-chewing high school football cheerleader.

TMDance. Intricate footwork performed by dentists who have just completed a big case on a pa-tient, and the patient is now complaining of jaw joint pain, and pretreatment records are sparse to nonexistent.

TMDaredevil. A dentist who carries out definitive treatment on a patient with symptomatic joints.

TMDark-ages. We're in them.

TMDasher. A dentist who dashes (as, into treatment without a diagnosis).

TMData. Collected by those interested in an accurate diagnosis.

TMDazzle. Witnessed by many dentists at weekend courses advertised in nationally distributed fliers.

TMDeadend. A position that offers no hope of progress. A fate common to two groups: 1) dentists who treat without a sound diagnosis; 2) their patients.

TMDeadwood. Useless and burdensome persons or things: Characterizing the view many dentists have of their patients who have "TMJ."

TMDebacle. Similar to TMDeadend except more extreme. In this case the patient gets worse.

TMDebate. A spectacle endemic to most professional meetings of dentists. A major form: those who say occlusion is the major factor in TM joint dysfunction and head pain, versus those who say TM patients are all crazier than loons. Both sides are wrong.

TMDebility. The state of being weak or feeble; weakness. Current status of knowledge of most TMDentists (if not all).

TMDebris. The ruins of anything broken down or

*Reprinted with permission from the *Journal of the California Dental Association*, 19(6):57–60, 1991.

destroyed; rubbish. 1) Plastic implants after removal from the joints. 2) What's left of the joints.

TMDecay. To decline in excellence, prosperity, health, etc.; deteriorate. An unfortunately accurate description of a few patients who have become destitute in repeated unsuccessful attempts to find help for their TM problems.

TMDecency. A quality shared by three groups. 1) Dentists who diagnose and treat their patients thoughtfully and conservatively; 2) patients who understand a major portion of the responsibility for success in treatment rests on their own shoulders; and 3) insurance companies who forswear obstructive claims payment policies.

TMDecimation. What happened to most of the joints subjected to artificial disc replacements.

TMDecor. Interior decoration of the mouth. Many colors, styles and variations. Mostly plastic, mostly worn on the teeth.

TMDecorum. Propriety of behavior, speech, dress, etc. As with decorum in general, context is a crucial determinant. Some examples of proper TMDdecorum:

Context	Behavior
TMDemagogue with **DMDisciples**	Authoritative, omniscient, fatherly.
TMDisciples with **TMDemagogue**	Respectful, eager, appreciative, fully paid.
TMDisciples with **TMDupes**	Authoritative, omniscient, fatherly.
TMDupes with **TMDisciples**	Respectful, eager, appreciative, fully paid.

TMDecree. An ordinance or edict promulgated by a TMDemagogue. *Syn:* TMDictum.

TMDefault. Similar to the computer term ("default") meaning "the standard value used in the absence of another choice." Dentists usually have a default splint. In fact very few can make more than one kind.

TMDefect. May apply to any of the following: 1) An actual physical problem in a TM joint; 2) a TMDisciple who is ready to treat patients after one weekend course; 3) the evidence upon which a TMDemagogue bases his approach to treatment.

TMDeference. Respectful, courteous regard. The way TMDemagogues want to be treated by TMDisciples.

TMDeficit. Shortage, deficiency. A descriptive term applicable to the current status of scientific knowledge of the pathophysiology of TMDisorders.

TMDegeneration. Also called DJD (degenerative joint disease). A process by which tissue degenerates. Particularly changes in the TM condyle with a characteristic radiographic appearance. Feared by many patients who have been warned by TMDisciples that it is inevitable if they don't agree to _____ therapy (fill in the blank with the TMDisciple's pet appliance, surgical procedure, etc.) Probably many people die of old age without ever knowing they had severe DJD in both joints.

TMDeity. Secret ambition of every TMDemagogue.

TMDejavu. What the patient experiences when told the other joint needs surgery.

TMDelicatessen. Multidisciplinary clinic.

TMDeliverance. Referral to a qualified TMDentist.

TMDelusion. A fixed, dominating or persistent false mental conception resistant to reason. For example, the patient who says: "Don't tell me about it, just fix it, Doc."

TMDemagogue. A person, esp. an orator, who gains power and popularity by arousing the emotions, passions, and prejudices of the people. Especially effective in teaching dentists about TMDisorders. Usually characterized by a religious zeal for a particular type of appliance (splint) which is reputed to have magical properties and is named after the TMDemagogue. May also apply to others who have equipment to sell (see listing under TMDoodad). Also see TMDisciple.

TMDementia. Mental deterioration, esp. when due to physical causes. Mostly found in TMDentists who tried to limit their practice to the treatment of TMDisorders. Proximate cause: Compulsive head pounding on the wall.

TMDemolition. The act or an instance of demolishing. 1) What some dentists do to patients. 2) What some patients do to dentists.

TMDemon. A TMDemagogue as seen by another TMDemagogue.

TMDentist. A dentist who accepts referrals for patients with TMDisorders. Foolishly, the original idea was based on the grievous error that a pot of restorative gold lay at the end of the rainbow. Most dentists who stick with it, after discovering their mistake, are independently wealthy, overtreating their patients, or poverty-stricken. It's not pretty.

TMDependency. Implies a dependent need for a TM. Silly word. Who doesn't need a TM?

TMDeposition. A statement under oath, taken down in writing, to be used in court. Vehicle used by TMDemagogues to further their own particular brand of TMDogma. TMDepositions are also given by honest TMDentists who attempt to help the court arrive at the truth. Sometimes it's tricky to know which is which.

TMDepravity. Perversion, corruption, debauchery; debased, degenerate; dissolute, profligate; licentious, lascivious, lewd, immoral. Not related to TMDisorders. Included here because the words are so luscious.

TMDepradation. To plunder or lay waste to; pillage; ravage. What people do to each other too often. For examples see TMDemagogue, TMDisciple and TMDevil.

TMDepression. Dejection, sadness, gloom. 1) The way a patient feels after months or years of unsuccessful treatment. 2) The way a dentist feels who has just been handed a summons from the patient in definition 1.

TMDerangement. Disarrangement, disorder. Term applied to 1) dysfunctional discs and 2) to dentists who treat TM problems without the benefit of diagnosis, or clearly defined treatment goals.

TMDerring-do. Daring deeds; heroic daring. *Syn:* TMDaredevil.

TMDesert. Wasteland, wilderness, arid. Supporting few lifeforms. The TM healthcare system as seen by a frustrated TM patient.

TMDesign. The Holy Grail of splint design as revealed through spiritual communication from On High to the TMDemagogue. *Unexplained curiosity:* Several exist but not all are the same even though they came from the same Source.

TMDestroyer. To injure beyond repair or renewal. Nothing can withstand this force. TM joints, teeth, dental work, splints all succumb. Fearsome. Dentists tremble in its presence. *Syn:* Bruxer.

TMDetour. Roundabout or circuitous way or course. Experienced commonly by patients who go to a TMDisciple who tries to cure migraine headaches by fixing the patient's occlusion.

TMDevil. The author of this dictionary. A striking case of arrested development as revealed by the juvenile humor.

TMDevotee. 1) A patient (slightly out of date) who still thinks it's fashionable to have "TMJ." 2) (*rare*) A dentist who actually studies the pathophysiology of TMDisorders with an open mind.

TMDiagnosis. (*rare*) The act of determining in advance of treatment the exact nature of the patient's problem using data gathered from a thorough history, clinical examination and imaging. Major advantage (widely unappreciated): Ability to individualize treatment for each patient to maximum benefit.

TMDialectic. A dialectic is an argumentation or discussion based on logic, as of the truth of a theory or opinion. The TM variant is exceedingly rare. Its existence is postulated mainly on theoretical grounds since there is no known reason it could not exist. Occasional reports of rare sightings. No actual witnesses known.

TMDiatribe. A bitter, abusive denunciation. The most common form of communication among various groups purporting interest in TMDisorders. However, among dentists in general it ranks a distant second place to apathy.

TMDictionary. A subversive document containing occasional moments of honesty.

TMDictum. An authoritarian pronouncement. See TMDemagogue. Variant of the more general dental dicta commonly found in all dental schools. *Syn:* TMDogma.

TMDiehard. A person who vigorously maintains or defends a hopeless position, outdated attitude, lost cause. Characterizes all TMDemagogues and TMDisciples. *Pathognomonic sign:* Knows how to make only one kind of splint (thought to have originally been handed down to Moses with the Ten Commandments) and uses it on every patient.

TMDiet. A particular selection of food from blenders.

TMDilemma. A situation requiring a choice between equally undesirable alternatives. Any difficult or perplexing situation or problem. Esp. common among TMDisciples with expensive equipment and lucrative reconstruction practices who learn through objective study that they may have been overtreating their patients.

TMDilettante. A person who takes up an art, activity, or subject merely for amusement. Most common among dentists who have several million hours of continuing education credits from all over the country.

TMDiploma. A document given by an educational institution. Used by TMDemagogues to legitimize their dogma. Comforting to TMDisciples who want to feel "in the know" with minimal expenditure of effort. Impressive to patients who see them on the walls of TMDisciples.

TMDisability. A golden prize sought after by patients who haven't won the lottery, but close inspection reveals that the term applies more aptly to the dentists who don't know what they're doing.

TMDisaffection. Feeling found in patients who, after the expenditure of multiple thousands of dollars, still have their problem.

TMDisappearance. 1) What some dentists at serious scientific courses on TMDisorders manage to do after they have gotten the course number for licensure renewal. 2) Condylolysis.

TMDisaster. A calamitous event, esp. one occurring suddenly and causing great damage or hardship, as in the discovery that a great many patients *need no treatment* other than some thoughtful education.

TMDisc. Where the action is. Splendid source of revenue to TMDisciples who attempt to recapture it and to surgeons who 1) arthroscope it; 2) plicate it; and 3) remove it.

TMDiscard. A patient whose disc has been 1) recaptured; 2) arthroscoped; 3) plicated; and 4) removed.

TMDisciple. A pupil or adherent of another. A goldmine for the bank accounts and the egos of TMDemagogues. Convinced of the sanctity of the "(name of TMDemagogue)-splint." Intensive study indicates that the TMDisciple was born with a potential capacity to think for himself, but this was effectively squelched in dental school.

TMDiscord. Two TMDemogogues lecturing at the same meeting.

TMDiscourse. To give forth, talk; a form of oratory. Characterizing the normal mode of communication of TMDemagogues—both on and off stage. Musical to their own ears.

TMDiscovery. 1) (*common*) The creative imaginings of TMDemagogues. 2) (*rare*) A scientifically sound study published in a respectable journal. 3) (*exceedingly rare*) A meaningful, scientifically sound study published in a respectable journal.

TMDisdain. How some insurance companies treat patients with serious need for care.

TMDisease. A condition of the body in which there is incorrect function resulting from heredity, infection, diet, or environment and for which afflicted persons seek treatment which is occasionally successful. Most of the time they recover better if they avoid treatment.

TMDisfigurement. Most prominent feature of a subset of post-surgical patients. See TMDiscard.

TMDisgrace. The state of being in dishonor; ignominy; shame, as when a TMDisciple renounces the sanctity of the TMDemagogue's TMDogma and admits he or she was wrong.

TMDislocation. 1) The translation of the mandibular condyle(s) anteriorly of the summit of the articular eminence. Reduction may require medical assistance. 2) What happens to patients when they receive the bill of the TMDemagogue.

TMDisorder. Any of a group of related maladies, conditions, or dysfunctions having to do with the TMjoints, muscles of mastication and related structures. Internationally recognized classifications exist. May or may not be known to TMDisciples and TMDemagogues.

TMDissection. Cutting, opening, repairing or removing TM joint structures. Occasionally done for study in cadavers. Often done for profit in living patients.

TMDividend. That which accrues to certain TMDisciples who polish their lecturing skills and study to be TMDemagogues.

TMDivorce. In patients: one of the etiologic factors of TMDisorders. In dentists: An impossible fantasy regarding referral of certain of their TM patients elsewhere (esp. after treatment has commenced).

TMDoc. Slang for TMDentist.

TMDoctrine. A particular principle, position, or policy taught or advocated, as of a religion, etc. Advanced form of TMDogma (see listing). Key features: Must be taken on faith, may not be questioned and may be changed only by the TMDemagogue.

TMDogma. Subclassification of the more general term Dental Dogma. Any of a variety of unsubstantiated assertions propounded by TMDemagogues and dental school instructors. Very similar to TMDoctrine.

TMDolor. Sorrow; grief, anguish. How TM patients feel about their problems. How dentists feel about their TM patients.

TMDomicile. A place of residence. Normally the glenoid fossa, occasionally the cutting room floor.

TMDon. A person of great importance. A head, fellow, or tutor of a college. A TMDemagogue at a dental school.

TMDoodad. A decorative embellishment; trinket; bauble, gadget. As in fully adjustable articulators and electromyographic devices. To qualify for the "TM" prefix, they may cost in five figures. Very common application for the TMDoodad: substitute for thinking.

TMDotage. Feebleness of mind resulting from 1) hotel courses on TMDisorders; 2) too many TM patients in one day; or 3) returning to graduate school in midlife.

TMDowner. A depressing experience, person, or thing. *Often:* TM patients. *More often:* Dentists who try to treat TM patients.

TMDrifter. 1) A patient who, like Diogenes' search for one honest man, drifts from dentist to dentist searching for one who can help. 2) *Variant:* A patient who can't recognize a dentist able to help even if one were found.

TMDrugs. Overused by some, underused by others. Almost never used correctly.

TMDDuck. A movement made by many dentists when approached by a patient with a jaw joint problem. See TMDump.

TMDullard. Variant of dullard (a stupid person). A dentist who treats every TM patient the same way.

TMDump. The act of ridding oneself of something irresponsibly. The TMDump is a highly advanced form in which a treating dentist convinces unwanted TM patients of the remarkable expertise of dentist colleagues. *Syn:* referral, turfing.

TMDysfunction. Any of a number of actual physical problems affecting the TM joint. Poorly understood by most dentists.

TMDyspepsia. Deranged digestion resulting from having read this far.

THE EMPEROR'S NEW MENISCUS*

Edward B. Seldin, D.M.D., M.D.

With apologies to Hans Christian Andersen.

Once upon a time, in a land not unlike our own, there was a great period of inflation. This was a profound source of discomfiture to the Emperor who took the well-being of his subjects to heart. The Dow Jones Industrial Average had not yet been invented, but the number of furrows in the Emperor's brow was accepted as a reliable index of the state of the economy.

As if the economic woes of his realm were not enough, the Emperor developed a royal case of TMJ pain dysfunction syndrome. Actually, it was his good wife, the Empress, who made the diagnosis. She made it a practice to stay abreast of the latest trends in health care and remained in the vanguard of the medically well informed by reading such primary source material as *Reader's Digest* and *Time* magazine. Fortunately for the Emperor, there was an abundance of health care providers in the land. The problem was to choose just the right kind of practitioner to treat the royal pain. "Why not summon representatives of each discipline?" said the Empress; and that's exactly what they did.

When word got out that the Emperor was afflicted with a TMJ problem, there was great excitement amongst the health care providers. Most were motivated by a sincere desire to help the Emperor; but there were a few who recognized a chronic remunerative condition when they saw it. Here was the perfect way to "inflation-proof" their practices. And so, from far and near, experts flocked to the palace to minister to the Emperor.

There were general dentists, oral surgeons, periodontists, prosthodontists, and chiropractors. There were experts in occlusion, biofeedback, nutrition, and numerous other disciplines, all hoping that their modality of therapy would find favor with the Emperor.

Straws were drawn to see who would examine the Emperor first. A highly renowned expert on occlusion was selected. The Emperor underwent a full gnathologic assessment after which the first expert proclaimed, "No wonder His Majesty is in pain! His centric occlusion and centric relation are not in harmony. Moreover, there are gross prematurities and no balancing contacts in lateral excursion. What the Emperor needs is a program of occlusal equilibration."

This sounded good to the Emperor who, being evenhanded by nature, agreed to undergo equilibration. Not wanting to be guilty of favoritism, the Emperor called upon other experts who instituted megavitamin therapy and a diet low in sucrose. He also had his spine adjusted and wore an occlusal appliance to prevent bruxism. Electrodes were attached to the royal crown to record alpha waves, perform electromyography, and stimulate the muscles of mastication. Everyone marveled at how well the Emperor adhered to the therapy despite the heavy demands of the Empire.

At the end of the course of therapy, the Emperor had to admit that he was much better. However, it is unbecoming of an Emperor to be better, even much better—an Emperor must be Best. And, besides, none of the conservative modes of treatment had succeeded in preventing painful dislocation of the Royal TMJ. This occurred almost every time he protruded his lower jaw, which he did frequently to add gravity to his pronouncements and because he was a secret admirer of Henry VIII.

After much discussion it was agreed that only arthrography would fully elucidate the Emperor's problem. His Majesty could only bow to the collective wisdom of the experts and arthrograms were done.

*Reprinted with permission by the ADA Publishing Co., Inc., from the *Journal of the American Dental Association*, 106:615–616, 1983.

"No wonder the Emperor is still symptomatic," exclaimed the royal arthrographer. "He has internal derangement of the TMJ." No one had ever seen a royal arthrogram before and it took a while for the significance of this study to register. Soon it became clear to all that the Emperor must either live with his affliction or undergo surgery. The Emperor, for his part, was secretly glad that the X rays showed something. He was worried that the problem was all in his head and it was good to have it confirmed that an actual physical problem existed.

Inexorably, the day of surgery approached. When it arrived, all activity in the Empire stopped and the populace maintained a vigil.

In the operating room a team of surgeons approached the royal TMJ via a standard preauricular incision. When, in due course, the capsule was exposed, it was clear to all that there was herniation of the meniscus. However, it was less clear in which direction this had occurred. Some thought lateral, others thought anterior, still others were convinced it was posterior.

A heated debate then ensued as to the type of correction to apply. There were calls for menisectomy, with and without Silastic implant. There were advocates of condylectomy, condylotomy, and condylar shave. Some thought strongly that his eminence should be removed, but it was quickly pointed out that this might be misinterpreted as a symbolic act in support of separation of church and state. The Emperor's surgeons knew better than to mix surgery and politics.

After much discussion it was decided that a high condylectomy was best suited to the lofty personage of the Emperor and a meniscus plication was added for good measure.

As he recovered from surgery, the Emperor was not exactly sure how he felt. But at this point he had a totally different perspective on the significance of his presenting symptoms. His Majesty found it expedient to report that he indeed felt well. As Emperor, one zealously defends the credibility of one's appointees.

When, at last, the Emperor held his first postoperative public audience, the people marveled at how well he looked. It did not escape notice that His Majesty's brow (or at least half of it) was entirely free of furrows. News of this encouraging sign spread far and wide. This ushered in a period of economic recovery and a level of prosperity previously unknown in the realm.

For their part, the Emperor's surgeons were happy that they had successfully returned His Majesty to the state of health that he had enjoyed before surgery. The Emperor showed his gratitude to his experts by creating for them a Royal TMJ Institute and by decreeing that their practices be limited to the treatment of TMJ pain dysfunction syndrome.

The moral of this tale is that treating TMJ disorders is like looking for a restaurant in an unfamiliar town: it's hard to know which joint to enter and which one to stay out of. So when your own disk is at risk, choose carefully whom you appoint to treat your joint.

ANDROCLES AND THE (RICH) LION . . . AN UPDATE*

Stewart Whitmarsh, D.D.S.

Dr. Stewart Whitmarsh is the former editor of the Journal of the Colorado Dental Association.

In order to fully appreciate the New Age in which we practice, one has to be able to read and understand the New Age Revised Fables. One of them relates the tale of the Androcles and the Rich Lion.

Not so long ago, a young man named Androcles set up shop in a cave. A Rich Lion, passing by, said: "Please help me, for I am in great distress." Now Androcles, being a brave if somewhat dull-witted young man, invited the Rich Lion into his cave so he could "take a look."

The Rich Lion pointed to a thorn stuck between his teeth (central incisors, #8 and #9), and said, with a pleading look on his face, "I would give *anything* to have the pain relieved." Androcles, not one to miss a vital clue since reading a journal article entitled, "Adding Tons of Cash to Your Paycheck," asked, "Anything?" The Rich Lion, realizing that Androcles might be smarter than he looked, replied: "Anything . . . within a reasonable limit."

Now, you have to understand that, although Androcles had the IQ of a Rhesus monkey, it was augmented by a totally avaricious outlook on life. He had been told by his therapist that this characteristic was certainly not a flaw and most likely the result of 1) his dysfunctional family, 2) low self-esteem, 3) the school system, and was "even an attribute in this materialistic world." That his therapist was a Democrat and a closet, but very confused, Rush Limbaugh wannabe was unknown to Androcles.

To further update this fable, Androcles had just sat through a seven-hour seminar (". . . Interested in doubling your income?") presented by a renowned entrepreneur who was raking in more on the lecture tour than he had ever been able to produce in his office. He had thoroughly researched two cases to support his seven-hour lecture (". . . lunch included") on Thorn Removal (TR^R).

"What a lucky day," Androcles said to himself. "Not only for this very Rich Lion—but for me!"

He addressed the Lion in a professional manner, thusly: "Mr. Lion, you do indeed have a serious problem here, and it is fortunate for you that I have just completed an extensive seminar in alternative skills and have acquired knowledge that the other thorn removers lack." He smiled and added, "And naturally, there is a higher fee involved, as I am a Specialist in TR^R."

He went on to explain: "Modern TR^R depends on a holistic non-traditional approach, which will balance your body chemistry and bring it into harmony with nature. Today, we not only diagnose and treat TR^R with surface electromyography sonography, but with Doppler ultrasound, thermography and electronic stimulation. In Advanced TR^R, I advocate orthomolecular psychiatry tuned to your deeper psychic self, applied kinesiology, auriculo-therapy, cranical osteopathy and various blends of herbology, homeopathy, naturopathy, iridology . . . and even, Mr. Lion, *Divine intervention*." Androcles bowed his head, with a suitably ecclesiastical look, hoping the situation would not get that desperate.

"It will also be necessary," Androcles continued, "to provide you with some edible detoxifying supplements ('. . . before and following removal'), a special nostrum to enhance your particular energy flow, and an irrigation solution, composed of two natural ingredients 'keyed' to your periodontopathic bacteria. All of these things I am able to sell you right here in this cave, for a small additional

*Reprinted with permission from the *Journal of the Colorado Dental Association*, 73(Oct):9–10, 1994.

DISEASE, PATHOLOGY, AND RESEARCH (AND OTHER THINGS IN JOURNALS)

cost. I accept discount coupons, all of the usual credit cards and give a 5% discount for cash. Please sign this 23-page waiver and disclaimer form."

The Rich Lion was awed. He signed and gladly forked over the money, which was far in excess of the UCR for TR[R]. Androcles removed the thorn from between the central incisors (#8 and #9) in 25 seconds flat. The Rich Lion went on his way, a happier lion . . . until, later on, several problems were discovered in another cave down the street.

Unfortunately, Androcles had missed a field of rampant caries, parsecs of pockets (Rich Lions have deep pockets) and another thorn between the Rich Lion's bicuspids (#20 and #21) which was the real source of infection.

Time passed. But not so much time that the Statute of Limitations was exceeded. A letter addressed to Androcles arrived from a well-known TV attorney ("Are you getting all you should get from your injury?"), accusing Androcles of fraud, chicanery, charlatanism and other nasty things—and demanding 2.5 mil.

That the case was settled out of court for considerably less did little to mollify Androcles. "It seems to me there was a time when lions were grateful for what we did for them," complained Androcles. "What's happening in this New Age today?"

Moral: In this mixed up, upside down New Age, don't expect solutions if you are part of the problem. . .

DENTISTRY, THE LAW, AND REGULATION

How many of us wish that we had invested in latex-producing companies 10 years ago? Fifteen years ago, I thought that OSHA was the sound that a washing machine made during the rinse cycle. Times change; we change.

I WAS A TEENAGE HAZARDOUS MEDICAL WASTE GENERATOR*

Andrew P. Tanchyk, D.M.D.

I tried not to admit to the vague sense of guilt and paranoia, or to a slight uptick in pulse and blood pressure. I am a professional, and I would stay focused and be sharp as I treated Mrs. Wills' root canal.

In my office was a young lad from the DEP. That's Department of Environmental Protection for non-doctors. For by now, in addition to learning all the traditional basic medical and clinical sciences, every medical and dental student has learned the meaning and importance of the DEP, EPA, OSHA and dozens of other wonky government and bureaucratic rules, regulations, requirements, standards, laws and mandates. He was a courteous lad, three years out of one of the state schools which produce the gears that manage most of our state's bureaucracies and hotels. His scrubbed appearance reminded me of one of the young deacons in my church.

I knew there was no reason I should feel any surge in my paranoia or pulse. After all, he had been here before, in 1992. And everything was OK, sort of.

"Everything is OK? Well everything is here, Doc . . . it just could be a little more organized, a little neater. Can I make a suggestion?"

Sure I can take it. I mean I think neatness and organization is important when I'm doing root canals and extractions. I just never got around to it with my DEP logs.

What was happening here was that a few of a drug addict's needles were found on some New Jersey beach during the 1988 elections. It was clear to the politicians that the best way to make the republic's beaches safe was to have every doctor in the state spend several hundred dollars and take a few dozen hours a year weighing their hazardous wastes and filling out forms, and to submit to audits by DEP inspectors to confirm that the doctors are in compliance with whatever law had been passed.

Most doctors I knew disposed of needles in separate receptacles anyway. How the paperwork and audits reduced the presence of addicts' needles on beaches was never stated. Doctors now had a new black hat to wear—Hazardous Medical Waste Generators (doctors have been addressed as "Dear Regulated Medical Waste Generator" by the DEP in some correspondences).

There were also many incongruities. A diaper or extracted tooth disposed of in a doctor's office was hazardous medical waste. They had to be weighed, registered on a log and quadruplicate tracking form, and then transported, treated, and destroyed by an EPA or DEP approved transporter, treater and destroyer. If the patient brought them home they were just garbage. Tommy Crowley could take home his extracted baby tooth and put it under his pillow or throw it at his sister and it was now cute rather than hazardous.

It was also confusing when the government and bureaucracy that was always telling us to lower health care costs was always raising them with another rule, regulation, requirement, standard, law, mandate, tax or fee.

However, bureaucracy is persistent in its commandments and taboos. Doctors want to be perceived by themselves and other as good guys/gals. So it wasn't long till I noted in me and all of my colleagues vague feelings of guilt and the need for repentance. In fact there was a new awareness of not only our own sins but those of others. We no longer looked at just our offices but all of society—restaurants, hair salons, rest rooms, everything—as hazardous medical waste generation units, occasions of sin! The only salvation for our own sins was to do our bureaucratic penance.

*Reprinted with permission from the *Journal of the New Jersey Dental Association*, (Winter): 71–73, 1995.

Playing It by Ear

I admit at the beginning with the DEP paperwork I was sort of faking it. We'd never been taught this in school. That is what Howard (my own physician) and I admitted to one another at my annual check up in 1990. What the hell are you doing with all this OSHA and DEP crap? he asked me. I'm sort of playing it by ear, kind of faking it till I know what's going on, I answered. He smiled and said he was doing the same thing. He clearly felt better that I wasn't too far ahead of him on the policy wonk curve.

It was about then that a bit of heresy entered my consciousness. He was about to listen to my heart and lungs and check my hemorrhoid, when I thought, as a patient, do I want my doctor spending his time and money complying with the DEP? Or, spending his time and money taking a course or reading a book about hearts or lungs or hemorrhoids? Even for me. Mrs. Will might benefit someday on the course they give at Penn on advanced root canal treatments.

The most attended courses in recent years by physicians and dentists have not been on hearts, hemorrhoids or root canals, but courses that teach doctors how to comply with bureaucratic rules, regulations, requirements, standards, laws and mandates.

In fact, I was ready to say that Howard should use the extra time and money on himself and relax a little. In addition to all the other pressure on my doctor, did I really want him worrying about being labeled a *Hazardous Medical Waste Generator?* Would it change my opinion of him if he was cited for a DEP violation?

Surely there is some wisdom in the discipline of the monthly weighing of one pound of needles that we generate or the organizational abilities of keeping our DEP papers orderly or the neatness and accuracy of filling in with a number two pencil the annual DEP Waste Generator Report. These thoughts drifted from my consciousness when he reported that my heart, lungs and hemorrhoid would survive another year.

The suggestion the DEP lad made to me on his first visit in 1992 was a *deja vu.* "What I'd like you to do, Doc, is get one of those one-inch soft-cover loose-leaf binders. Do you know the ones I mean?" Indeed I did! "And you can get folders that fit into it. Do you know the ones I mean." I did, I really did!

"Label one folder Monthly Logs." I interrupted him, grabbed a piece a paper and took notes. He seemed pleased at that, not only I suppose, because I was being compliant to my superiors in the bureaucracy (why should I make a fight out of this I thought, it's not worth the time or energy), but also I sensed the glee in him that a boring teacher has when all the brown-nosing students studiously take notes of the lecture.

"First folder—monthly logs. Second folder—tracking form receipts. Third folder—annual reports. Fourth folder—generator ID number and DEP correspondence. Fifth folder—miscellaneous." Then came the *coup de grace.* "If you do this, doc, you'll also be in compliance with the federal OSHA regulations on medical waste." My God! A bureaucratic twofer. There was a beauty and elegance in it all. As much as me doing a root canal or Howard removing a hemorrhoid.

Deja Vu All Over Again

The *deja vu* I had was from my annual September rite. Since kindergarten, every September, my three kids each bring home a list from school for assorted tablets, notebooks, binders and pens that each teacher requires. Sure enough, when I returned home that night, under a pile of crayons my 14-year-old daughter found an extra maroon-colored, one-inch, soft-covered loose-leaf binder. The lad from DEP had mentioned no specific color requirement for the binder, and maroon seemed like a professional color. Our family bible was maroon colored. In addition, we had several tan folders that would fit into the binder.

I read aloud from my crib sheet what the DEP lad suggested. As I raised my eyes, my daughter had already organized and labeled the binder and folders. Why not? She'd been doing it since kindergarten!

I was excited now and returned with my daughter to my office. In the time it took for me to check and answer my phone messages, she had neatly filled each folder with the correct paperwork in the proper alphabetical or numerical order. I picked up the binder and opened it like a high priest with a sacred text.

As a final touch I had my daughter scroll the title in black across the cover—**<u>Regulated Medical Waste Compliance.</u>** In the lower right-hand corner, in blue, she inscribed my name and Waste Generator ID number.

I faded back to 1994 and Mrs. Wills. I gave her postoperative instructions for her root canal, took a deep breath, and went back to the DEP lad in my office. He looked up and smiled. "Everything is OK doc, you're in compliance." I was in compliance! The Lord Be With You!

When the DEP lad left, I placed my right hand on the binder. I felt embarrassed at first for my prior immaturity and rebelliousness. I had been like a teenager faking a final exam. Now it was all becoming clear.

I had a perverse wish that my hemorrhoid flare up so I could share with Howard my new knowledge and acceptance. I felt more mature, more professional.

I thought of my daughter. How proud I was that she had this opportunity! To learn, at such a young age, that in the real world being a doctor was not just about root canals and hemorrhoids—but maroon, one-inch, soft-covered loose-leaf binders with tan folders!

POLITICALLY CORRECT DENTIST*

Harriet Seldin, D.M.D.

In the politically correct 90s, the old ways of thinking just don't work. Whether in the legislative arena or their own offices, politically correct dentists must learn how to behave.

"Independence," as in "independent practice for hygienists," sounds politically correct. Issues of "undiagnosed care" or "unsupervised practice" don't even enter into the picture. A "single standard of care" doesn't mean a thing. Organized hygiene is benefiting from the politically correct interest in the underdog.

The (California) Assembly recently passed AB 221, the independent practice hygiene bill, along with several other seemingly unrelated pieces of legislation. AB 2020, a bill to allow optometrists to prescribe therapeutic drugs, was passed out of the Health Committee and the Ways & Means Committee. AB 671, sponsored by the California Association of Oral and Maxillofacial Surgeons (and supported by CDA), relating to nondiscrimination toward joints, was also passed by the Health Committee. The bill would require insurance carriers to cover the TMJ more like a knee.

What do these bits of legislation have in common? The interests of the underdog. It's hygienist vs. dentist. Optometrist vs. ophthalmologist. Dentists vs. big bad insurance industry (also a touch of dentistry vs. medicine). In politically correct thinking, it all makes sense, even to the mentally challenged.

How does the politically correct dentist behave in his/her office? This is of critical importance considering the potential legal morass of sexual harassment, wrongful termination and the Americans with Disabilities Act. (It is unfortunate that the politically correct Americans with Disabilities Act shares an acronym with our own ADA. However, in politically correct society, it is acceptable to be confused, or factually challenged.)

The astute dentist does not speak of "decay" or "cavities." This sort of language is old-fashioned and politically incorrect. The proper terminology is "bacterially impaired" or "structurally disintegrated."

A staff member who shows up late for work is chronologically deficient. A patient who can't fit into your dental chair is horizontally enhanced. As a female dentist, I must be gender-sensitive to male pattern behavior, such as the position of the unisex office toilet seat.

If, by some unfortunate circumstances, an OSHA employee chooses to visit your office, please respond in a politically correct manner. Instead of requesting a search warrant for the OSHA rep to enter your office, why not inform him that you are regulation-challenged? If that's good enough for the U.S. Department of Health and Human Services (with politically correct Donna Shalala in charge), this answer should be good enough for you.

Offer to show the OSHA inspector around your politically correct office. In Operatory 1, your patient, a female combat pilot's domestic partner (sexual preference unknown), covered under spousal dental benefits for TMJ treatment, is having an impression of her upper dental arch. Is anything wrong with this picture? Is everything autoclaved?

In Operatory 2, a child who is legally divorced from his parents needs an occlusal restoration. You're not sure whose consent you must obtain before starting the procedure, but that should not be relevant to the OSHA inspector. That is, not unless a receptionist gets a paper cut from the consent form, or any indecent proposals are overheard on the office intercom.

In Operatory 3, an optically under-achieving patient wishes to have microabrasion for those unsightly white spots on his maxillary laterals. He just came from his optometrist's office, and is having trouble focusing with his dilated pupils. It's not your fault that he knocked over the properly la-

*Reprinted from *CDA Update,* July 19, 1993, with permission of the California Dental Association.

beled hydrofluoric acid and burned holes through your chair and carpet. Since no staff members were injured (and all are wearing longsleeved lab coats and goggles), the inspector shouldn't be too concerned.

However, to distract the inspector, you suggest that he visit your neighbor, a visually impaired hygienist who has recently set up his laser soft tissue management practice next door. You're not sure if all the secondary containers for mouthwash and prophy paste are labeled in braille.

The OSHA inspector won't care that your latex gloves are destroying the rain forest. He won't mind that the air conditioner in the car that takes your case to the lab is poking holes in the ozone layer. But you'll care and be reassured that purity of thought has been reestablished and your conscience is politically correct.

LATEX*

Donald F. Bowers, D.D.S.

Latex is a friend of mine,
I wear it every day.
It fits so snug upon my hands,
And keeps viruses away.

With latex to protect me,
I practice without a care.
Except the damn things cost me
Thirty cents a pair.

*Reprinted with permission from the *Ohio Dental Journal,* (Winter):11, 1988.

THERE OUGHT TO BE A LAW!*

Some silly laws are on the books that affect dentists. One author, in researching city ordinances from across the country, discovered some real doozies. You have to wonder what events transpired to cause people to pass these laws.–Ed.

- It's against the law in Lignite, North Dakota, for a dentist to toss an old shoe at any woman who comes in for an appointment with her hair in rollers.

- In Slick Rock, Colorado, it's against the law for a dentist to wear a sock with a hole in the toe. (Who's checking?)

- In McCabe, Montana, no one cares about toe holes. An ordinance there specifies that no dentist can ever be seen in public places wearing socks with holes in the heels.

- An old law in Blue Earth, Minnesota, prohibits dentists from playing checkers during lunch hours.

- Only licensed dentists in Homer, Illinois, are legally allowed to tote a slingshot.

- If you practice in Point Comfort, Texas, you better smile. It's against the local law for a dentist to frown at a patient.

- In Hephzibah, Georgia, no patient can make faces at a dentist while teeth are being extracted. A patient who makes faces or even sticks his or her tongue out at a dentist can be fined $3.

- Lesterville, Missouri, dentists are prohibited from dipping snuff or even chewing tobacco while attending patients.

- In Rocky Mount, North Carolina, dentists who dip snuff in a public place can be slapped with a $5 fine or spend one night in the local jail.

- No female wearing a sheer nightgown in Round Spring, Missouri, can be legally treated by a local dentist. The law states that a woman of any age always must be fully attired before a dentist can assist her with an emergency. (What about the dentist?)

- In Buckhorn, New Mexico, criminals must "check all shooting irons" at the local dentist's office within 30 minutes after arriving in town. If the office is closed, the weapons must be left with the local physician.

- If a dentist in Bolivar, Ohio, takes part in a lynching, the community is liable to the victim for a sum of money "not to exceed" $500.

- No dentist practicing in Elk Mills, Maryland, is allowed to "lounge around" in an undershirt while working in the office.

- A dentist may not see patients while his or her breath "smells like wild onions" within the city limits of Toomsboro, Georgia.

- It's strictly against the law in Slaughter, Louisiana, for a dentist to allow a female patient to soak her feet while she sits in the waiting room.

*Reprinted with permission from the *Journal of the New Jersey Dental Association,* (Autumn):19, 1988.

COUNTERFEITED TOOTHBRUSHES CONFISCATED*

Nearly 180,000 counterfeit Colgate toothbrushes were destroyed and buried in the Franklin County Landfill in Columbus, Ohio. The counterfeit toothbrushes, which Colgate testing proved to be of inferior quality compared to genuine Colgate toothbrushes, were manufactured in Costa Rica and distributed to a major retailer in the East Central U.S. After Colgate brought suit, the retailer agreed to remove the counterfeit toothbrushes from the shelves of its over 200 outlets.

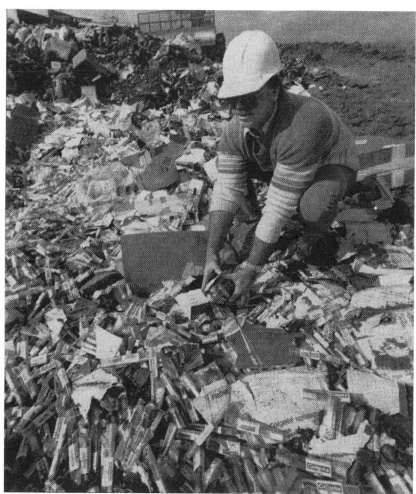

Pictured at the destruction site is Alfred Payne, manager, corporate security, Colgate U.S., who supervised the demolition of the counterfeit toothbrushes.

*Reprinted with permission from the *New York State Dental Journal*, (Jan):46, 1989.

DENTAL
HISTORY AND
DENTISTRY PAST

Dentists have been around for a long time. Our professional patriarch was a guy named Hesi-Re, who was described over 4,000 years ago by the Egyptian pharaoh Zoser as "the greatest of the physicians who treat the teeth". Undoubtedly, the first attempts at dental humor began the day after Hesi-Re started practice, and they have continued to this day.

RETURN OF THE WORM*

Donald F. Bowers, D.D.S.

One of the old theories of dental caries is the belief that tooth decay is caused by worms. The theory goes back to 12th-century Egypt and has been held in almost every civilization since then, including the ancient Sumerians, Greeks, Romans, Europeans, Chinese and American Indians. An old Japanese term for decayed tooth is *"mushi ba,"* or "worm tooth."

It is easy to see how the connection between tooth decay and worms has been made. From time immemorial, decayed meat has been associated with maggots and spoiled fruit with fruitworms. When wood rots, the process is marked by holes made by worms. When a tooth rots, there are holes observed in this process too; so, it seems reasonable to assume that worms might also be responsible for dental caries.

The "father of dentistry," Pierre Fauchard, was one of a number of notable European scientists who over the centuries looked for the elusive worm responsible for the condition that caused so much misery throughout the world. Antony Van Leeuwenhoek, the father of modern light microscopy, examined material from decayed teeth under his microscope and claimed to have seen worms that looked very much like creatures he had earlier identified in some old cheeses. Van Leeuwenhoek believed that foods were the source of tooth decay worms and established a theoretical link between caries and diet.

The worm theory of tooth decay persisted until the latter half of the 19th century when the new science of bacteriology emerged. When W. D. Miller formulated the bacteria–fermentable carbohydrate–acid–tooth decay theory in 1890, to which J. Leon Williams added the concept of plaque a few years later, the worm theory was placed on the shelf. After more than 3,000 years of acceptance, the theory disappeared from the literature, discarded *but never disproven.*

It seems to me that an idea which flourished for over 30 centuries deserves a better fate than it has received. After all, Miller's upstart chemoparasitic theory, a mere century old, is only a theory even though it forms the basis of modern cariology.

Who is to say that worms might not be the cause of dental caries just because there is a preponderence of scientific evidence to support another idea? I, for one, cannot turn my back on the works of such scientists and thinkers as the Roman Scribonius; the great European surgeon of the Middle Ages, Guy de Cahuliac; the 14th-century British priest-physician, Andrew Boorde; Fauchard; Van Leeuwenhoek and others.

But these are ancient characters who knew little about modern science, you say. So who built the pyramids, sailed across the Atlantic in a boat made of reeds, discovered oxygen without a spectrometer, determined that the earth is round and figured out how babies are made? The class of 1960? Of course not.

I argue for the worms. To hell with *S. mutans.* The major problem with the worm theory is that, with the exception of Van Leeuwenhoek, nobody has ever seen the culprits. The answer to that is easy. First of all, the worms are probably too small to be seen clinically, perhaps 10 microns or so in length. Secondly, I believe they live mostly in the blood stream and are photophobic. Therefore, they only emerge into the mouth when it is dark. The reason they have not been identified in blood smears is, again, their reaction to light. When the blood in which they reside is exposed to light, they curl up placing their tails in their mouths, forming a doughnut-shaped object similar to a miniature Cheerio, and look identical to a red blood cell under the microscope.

The worms only emerge at night to deposit their eggs (which microscopically resemble streptococci) in the plaque and eat away the enamel of teeth and

*Reprinted with permission from the *Ohio Dental Journal,* (Sep):9–10, 1984.

eventually reach the dentin which is their favorite food. Where do the worms come from? Van Leeuwenhoek was partially right. They come from food, but not fruits or cheese.

Tooth worms come from high-sugar food sources; sugar cane and bee's honey to name two, and from refined grains. That's why candy and cookies are bad for your teeth—not because of their effect on some silly, harmless bacteria that live in the mouth. (Incidentally, you can ask the chemoparasitic people this one: How is it that you can find *S. mutans* and the other so-called caries-causing bacteria in the mouths of caries-free people?) How does fluoride work to prevent tooth decay in respect to the worm theory, you ask? It's simple. Fluoride makes the enamel taste bad and the worms won't eat it.

Admittedly, the worm theory suffers from a lack of modern research data to support it. Unfortunately, the National Institutes of Health and the Research Institute of the American Dental Association are not at all eager to undertake or fund research projects to support this time-honored theory. Pity.

Treating Dental Caries by Eliminating the Worm

The most effective method of treating worm-caused tooth decay over the years has been eliminating the worms by fumigations. Henbane seeds, one of the standard ingredients of the fumigating concoction used by early practitioners, are not easy to come by. However, henbane seed can be substituted with scopolamine, an alkaloid of the henbane plant. Here is my formula, which I have found to be very effective in preventing cavities since I started using it over ten years ago. (I remember it was shortly after the Ohio Legislature passed the mandatory fluoridation law.)

Make a mixture of 450 grains of scopolamine, two teaspoons of Burpee's green onion seed, and three drops of tarragon vinegar. Place the mixture in the center of a Pyrex pie pan. Add two drops of charcoal starter fluid and ignite the mixture. When the flames die down, have the patient breath in the fumes and hold them in the mouth for one minute, being careful not to inhale. This procedure should be repeated once a month, but only under the supervision of a licensed dentist.

DENTISTRY PAST: TALES FROM THE '20s*

Dr. Louis J. Fazio

Over the years, I have enjoyed treating many patients in their 70s and 80s. Invariably, they have vivid memories of their dental experiences as children and young adults and they are willing to share these stories. And some of them are quite interesting.

Keep in mind these folks were born before television, antibiotics, electric appliances, frozen foods and plastics.

In their time, a closet was for clothes, not for coming out of. Bunnies were small rabbits. Hardware meant nails and screws; software did not exist. A nickel bought enough stamps to mail one letter and two post cards.

Some of these people readily admit that as children, they'd never heard of a dentist. Many only saw a dentist when they had a toothache or infection. One man remembered losing all his teeth as a child—three from a baseball, two from falling downstairs, and the rest from eating candy all day.

One woman believed dentists and patients had a different perception of pain. She believed pain was when you yelled or jumped because you were hurt. Her dentist said pain was only sensation. "The real pain," he told her, "is when you pay the bill."

Another patient recalled having a toothache as a young adult. She feared losing her teeth, so she went to a "higher-class dentist."

"We don't pull teeth anymore," the higher-class dentist said. "Now we just remove the nerve. It's brand new, known as root canal work. Today, I will bore a hole in your tooth and pull out the nerve." And so, he took the drill and began to grind. It felt like a blasting engine going through rock.

"Hey," the patient said, "that hurts."

"That's not the nerve, it's only the dentin," the dentist said. "I don't know what is wrong with that dentin, but this happens a lot. Not to worry."

The dentist kept drilling and the woman said she could see smoke coming out of her mouth and noticed a horrible burnt odor. She jumped and the dentist stopped and gave her some gas. He said this would make the nerve-pulling absolutely painless. The woman remembers letting out a scream and asking if he had pulled the nerve.

"Not at all," he said. "I only touched it." After a sleepless night, the patient had the tooth pulled the next morning by her regular dentist.

A neighbor told me his dentist story. It seems as a youngster, he suffered from periodontal disease. By the time he was 28, his dentist told him all his teeth needed to be removed because of "pyorrhea," which could not be treated.

Six months after the extractions, the patient was ready to have full dentures made.

"At the first appointment," my neighbor said, "the dentist put a plateful of plaster in my mouth. As I started to gag and wiggle, I was told to keep perfectly still. Several minutes passed, but it seemed like a week. The dentist started stabbing at my plaster with a knife because it wouldn't come out of my mouth.

"Finally the dentist yells 'It's out.' He looks at this chunk of caulk and frowns. 'A piece is missing,' he says. I'm afraid to tell him I swallowed it because he may go after it. 'Darn, we'll have to take another impression,' my neighbor continues.

"A month later, we're ready to try in the dentures. The dentist wants me to see and approve the teeth before the final denture is made. I arrive early one morning. After he puts the dentures in my mouth, he hands me a mirror. 'Look at these,' he said, 'if you want to make any changes, now is the time to do it. I'll be back, I need to make a phone call,' he told me.

"After 10 minutes, a young woman whom I had not seen before comes into the room," my neighbor said about his experience. "She tells me she is going to be a dental nurse and this is her first day. I asked her if she would bring me a cup of coffee while I'm waiting for the dentist to come back. Several minutes later, she brings my drink. I begin to sip the

*Reprinted with permission from *Today's FDA,* (Jan):5, 1995.

coffee slowly. Suddenly, I notice I have a mouthful of UFOs—unidentified floating objects. I sputter and spit. The dentist comes back into the room. 'What have you done to my wax try in? It took me a month to set those teeth!" He sees the cup of coffee and asks me where I got it.

"I saw the young woman about a week later at the corner grocery store and asked her how the job was going. She said, 'The job is gone. I'm selling oil-drilling equipment for a company in Texas. It's as close to a dental job as I could get.'"

Obviously, the dental profession has made great strides over the past 70 years.

Perhaps, in 70 years, someone will write an article on how dentistry was practiced around 2000. Those who read it may reflect on how primitive our practice standards were.

Let's hope so!

PREVENTION AND CURE OF TOOTHACHE*

Gardner P. H. Foley, M.A.

As long as there have been toothache and other painful oral troubles afflicting young and old, there have been folk remedies. The fact that many of these remedies were recorded in health books and "herbals" for several centuries would indicate that the recipients of the treatments had an enduring faith in their therapeutic values.

Being something of an antiquarian, I relish a work like *Brief Lives* by John Aubrey (1626–97). It is, at first thought, surprising that a man of Aubrey's stature would pay his respects to this bit of folklore:

> To cure the Tooth-ach, Take a new Nail, and make the Gum bleed with it, and then drive it into an Oak. This did Cure William Neal, Sir William Neal's Son, a very stout Gentleman, when he was almost Mad with the Pain, and had a mind to have Pistoll'd himself.

Obviously, then, the important point reflected is that the earnest acceptance of the therapeutic value of such a procedure was universal in Great Britain of the 17th century, not confined to the underprivileged majority.

In this sketch of "Sir John Birkenhead," Aubrey introduces other popular belief:

> I remember at Bristow (when I was a boy) it was a common fashion for the woemen to get a Tooth out of a Sckull in the Church yard; which they wore as a preservative of the Tooth-ach.

Perhaps there still lingers in parts of England the old faith in the superstition of preventing the toothache by clothing one's right leg prior to the left.

The writer of *A Rich Cabinet*, a curious book printed in 1668, refers to a belief that has had a wide circulation, both chronologically and geographically: "I have been certified (but how true it is I know not) that three teeth taken out of a dead man's skull and served in a clout or piece of leather, and worn about them which were subject to the toothache, it gave them present ease, and they never were troubled with the same so long as they had those about them."

An English dentist reported in 1875 on an unusual Egyptian practice: "One of the gates in Cairo is covered with portions of hair, clothing, etc., of those who have suffered, whilst into almost every crack and crevice carious teeth have been thrust, the idea prevailing that relief may be attained in this way."

William Butler Yeats, the great Irish poet, cites in his *Autobiographies* two unusual cures for the toothache:

> My father had a very black beard and hair, and one cheek bulged out with a fig that was there to draw the pain out of a bad tooth. One of the nurses said to the other that a live frog, she had heard, was best of all.

In *The Swimmer Manuscript* (1932), James Mooney reports a Cherokee folk method of preventing the toothache: "Never throw the remains of anything you have chewed (a quid of tobacco, the skin of an apple in which you have bitten, etc.) into the fire; else the fire will chew your teeth."

Immigrants to our country brought with them from their native countries many folklore beliefs that were generally adopted by at least the following American generation. Writing in 1886 of his patients in the 1830's and 1840's, Dr. L. W. Bristol, of Lockport, New York, recalled the "ignorance and superstition among the mass of people, relative to teeth." Often he was requested by a patient not to touch the extracted tooth, but to roll it up in paper. Curious as to what was to be done with the tooth, he was sometimes told that the patient was going to bore a hole in a sweet apple tree, put the tooth in the hole and

*Reprinted with permission from Foley GPH: *Foley's Footnotes*. Wallingford, PA, Washington Square East Publ., 1972, p 20–24.

then plug the hole up. He was told by others that they were going into the woods, where they would turn their back, take three steps and throw the tooth back over their head while saying "Good-bye to toothache." Still others were going to burn their extracted teeth and scatter the ashes to the four quarters of the earth and in that way get rid of the toothache. However, many of these superstitious patients subsequently returned for extractions. Dr. Bristol also recalled that one of the many never-on-Friday superstitions was that a dentist should not commence to make a set of teeth on a Friday.

———————

In many countries, especially Ireland, there are holy wells with a long history of healing those who follow traditional procedures. Often there is a holy tree overhanging the well to which the sufferers tie strings of beads, rags, or bits of clothing so that it may bear the burden of the suppliants' ailments. The ritual also includes walking round the well and making the sign of the cross with pebbles on certain stones that have been worn into grooves by the long observance of the ceremony. These wells are supposed to be particularly helpful for the cure of toothache. In Ireland the customary visiting time is the first Sunday of each quarter of the Celtic year.

———————

The Grandfathers (1964), by Contrad Richter, is well laden with folkways that still persisted in a Maryland mountain valley about 1915. When Grandfather Murdoch fell victim to a belting ache in his last surviving tooth, he and other members of his tribe began to consider the best cures for it. First of all, there was white mule to "licker it away." But no white mule could be found in the neighborhood. Other recommendations included the application of poultices of bread and vinegar, placing a fresh-butchered weasel skin to his jaw, with the bloody side against the jaw, biting on a coffin nail with the bad tooth, and, the surest remedy of all, urinating against the cheek. But a relative solved the immediate situation by providing Grandfather with enough whiskey to make him dead to the world. The next morning Grandfather was led to the blacksmith's, where that casual operator removed the tooth in a hilarious scene.

———————

Joseph Nelson, who taught school in the Ozark country, reported an unusual folk belief of that area. Gram Slocum had twenty-odd teeth extracted during one visit to a dentist. "She took them carefully as he removed them and brought them home with her lest someone get them and be able to work a meanness against her by having part of her body."

Nelson encountered an Ozarkian who had become disillusioned concerning the value of a treatment for the toothache, a mode of oral therapy firmly entrenched in the folklore of that backward area. "Don't let nobody tell you that a splinter off a lightnin'-struck tree is any he'p to a toothache. I reckon I've tried it thousands of times, jist in hope, and I was never done a bit of good."

———————

One of the most valuable and certainly one of the most interesting sources of information about the folklore of the teeth is the British *Notes and Queries*, published since 1849.

In response to a query about the use of charms for the cure of the toothache, a Roman Catholic priest submitted what he judged to be the original version of a popular incantation:

As Peter sat on a marble stone,
The Lord came to him all alone:
"Peter, what makes thee sit there?"
"My Lord, I am troubled with the tooth ache."
"Peter arise and go home;
And you, and whoever for my sake
Shall keep these words in memory,
Shall never be troubled with the toothache."
(May 4, 1850)

Often this poem and its variations were written on a piece of parchment and worn around the neck. Another charm also had wide acceptance: "In point of efficacy none are reckoned better than a tooth taken from the mouth of a corpse, which is then enveloped in a little bag, and hung around the neck." (June 15, 1850)

Many "recipes" for the cure and prevention of the toothache were submitted.

Pare your finger and toe-nails, wrap the parings carefully up in a small piece of paper. Make a slit in the bark of an ash tree; loosen the bark a little from the trunk, slip the small parcel under the bark, press the opening together again as closely as possible, and you will no more be troubled with toothache. (June 3, 1865)

POPE JOHN XXI*

Gardner P. H. Foley, M.A.

Peter Hispanus, born in Lisbon circa 1226, practiced medicine and surgery in Siena before his election as pope in 1276 (he also studied theology and philosophy at university in case you were wondering). Among several books he authored was The Treasure of Helth, a compilation of treatments for various ailments culled from the Greek, Roman, and Arabic knowledge as well as medieval folklore. In it he includes a chapter on cures "For the Tothake," as excerpted below. Pope John XXI died in 1277, only 8 months after his election, and remains the only dentist who ever became pope.—Ed.

- The causes—The sinews being very hot or cold or great quality of humors falling from the head to the gums.
- The signs—The pain is known well enough.

Remedies

If you wash your mouth once a month with the wine of the decoction of wertworte, thou shalt be healed of the toothache.

In a vehement ache put a little of the juice of yellow flag in thine ear on the side as thy ache is; it will a little grieve thee, but immediately thy toothache shall cease.

Put henbane seeds upon the coals and receive the smoke thereof into the teeth by gaping and holding thy mouth over it; it killeth the worm and assuageth the pain.

That thy teeth never ache, take the powder that cometh of filing an hart's bone, and let it steep in water in a new earthen pot and so put it into thy mouth where thy grief is.

The juice of chicory put into the ear or nostril that is on the contrary side to the grief taketh away utterly the toothache.

Steep the bark of a mulberry tree root in the juice of a cluster of grapes unto half, and wash thy mouth therewith, and thy teeth never shall ache.

Rub thy teeth often with a parsnip root, and it shall take away the worms in them and aching forever.

Against a strong pain steep violets in wine and hold them in thy mouth.

Pound two bulbs of garlic and tie it about thy arm on that side that the tooth acheth near to the hand; it draweth away all the pain.

The milk of wertworte baked in the bran of corn and put into the hole of the tooth breaketh the tooth.

Wash thy teeth with the water of the decoction of pomegranate flowers and put the powder of the said flowers into the tooth; it doth make the teeth fast and taketh away the ache by restraining the decay.

If the aching be exceeding painful put thereto opium tempered with the yolk of an egg halfboiled.

If the hollow tooth be filled with crow's dung it breaketh the tooth and taketh away the pain.

The juice of the root of dog fennel or of the herb thereof put into the hole of the tooth will not permit any worm to live therein.

Rue boiled in wine and laid in form of a plaster upon the pain in the gums by drying up the humor it taketh away the pain.

Put the powder of red coral in the hole of thy tooth and it will fall out by the root.

Celery root hung about thy neck doth allay the toothache.

Strawberry leaves chewed taketh away the toothache.

The body and fatness of a frog applied doth make an easy means to put out the teeth.

Let the gums be rubbed with the ashes of a dolphin tooth; the teeth are thereby greatly helped, or if they be only touched with the tooth itself.

*Reprinted with permission from Foley GPH: *Foley's Footnotes.* Wallingford, PA, Washington Square East Publ., 1972, pp 5–8.

TUSHMAKER'S TOOTHPULLER*

George H. Derby

George Horatio Derby (1824–1861), an Army officer, contributed humorous sketches to newspapers and magazines. These sketches were collected in two popular books: Phoenixiana *(1855) and* Squibob Papers *(1865). Derby wrote under the pseudonym John Phoenix.—G.P.H.F.*

For this and the following two papers, we are indebted to the great dental historian Gardner P. H. Foley, who was the Professor of Dental Literature and Dental History, Baltimore College of Dental Surgery. The three papers were part of a symposium honoring the centennial of the New York Dental Society in 1968.—Ed.

Dr. Tushmaker was never regularly bred as a physician or surgeon, but he possessed naturally a strong mechanical genius and a fine appetite; and finding his teeth of great service in the latter propensity, he concluded that he could do more good in the world, and create more real happiness therein, by putting the teeth of its inhabitants in good order, than in any other way; so Tushmaker became a dentist. He was the man that first invented the method of placing small cogwheels in the back teeth for the more perfect mastication of food, and he claimed to be the original discoverer of that method of filling cavities with a kind of putty, which, becoming hard directly, causes the tooth to ache so grievously that it has to be pulled, thereby giving the dentist two successive fees for the same job.

Tushmaker was one day seated in his office, in the city of Boston, Massachusetts, when a stout old fellow, named Byles, presented himself to have a back tooth drawn. The dentist seated his patient in the chair of torture, and, opening his mouth, discovered there an enormous tooth, on the right hand side, about as large, as he afterwards expressed it, "as a small Polyglot Bible." I shall have trouble with this tooth, thought Tushmaker, but he clapped on his heaviest forceps and pulled. It didn't come. Then he tried the turn-screw, exerting his utmost strength, but the tooth wouldn't stir.

"Go away from here," said Tushmaker to Byles, "and return in a week, and I'll draw that tooth for you, or know the reason why." Byles got up, clapped a handkerchief to his jaw, and put forth. Then the dentist went to work, and in three days he invented an instrument which he was confident would pull anything. It was a combination of the lever, pully, wheel and axle, inclined plane, wedge and screw. The castings were made, and the machine put up in the office, over an iron chair rendered perfectly stationary by iron rods going down into the foundations of the granite building.

In a week old Byles returned; he was clamped into the iron chair, the forceps connected with the machine attached firmly to the tooth, and Tushmaker, stationing himself in the rear, took hold of a lever 4 feet in length. He turned it slightly. Old Byles gave a groan and lifted his right leg. Another turn; another groan, and up went the leg again. "What do you raise your leg for?" asked the doctor. "I can't help it," said the patient. "Well," rejoined Tushmaker, "that tooth is bound to come out now."

He turned the lever clear round with a sudden jerk, and snapped old Byles's head clean and clear from its shoulders, leaving a space of 4 inches between the severed parts!

They had a *post-mortem* examination—the roots of the tooth were found extending down the right side, through the right leg, and turning up in two prongs under the sole of the right foot! "No wonder," said Tushmaker, "he raised his right leg." The jury thought so too, but they found the roots much decayed; and five surgeons swearing that mortification would have ensued in a few months,

*Reprinted with permission from Foley GPH: Dentistry and the 19th century American humorists. *New York Journal of Dentistry*, 38(10):439–440, 1968.

Tushmaker was cleared on a verdict of "justifiable homicide."

He was a little shy of that instrument for some time afterward; but one day an old lady, feeble and flaccid, came in to have a tooth drawn, and thinking it would come out very easy, Tushmaker concluded, just by way of variety, to try the machine. He did so, and at the first turn drew the old lady's skeleton completely and entirely from her body, leaving her a mass of quivering jelly in the chair! Tushmaker took her home in a pillowcase. She lived 7 years after that, and they called her the "India-Rubber Woman." She had suffered terribly with the rheumatism, but after this occurrence, never had a pain in her bones. The dentist kept them in a glass case.

After this, the machine was sold to the contractor of the Boston Customhouse, and it was found that a child of 3 years of age could by a single turn of the screw, raise a stone weighing 23 tons. Smaller ones were made on the same principle, and sold to the keepers of hotels and restaurants. They were used for boning turkeys.

There is no moral to this story whatever, and it is possible that the circumstances may have become slightly exaggerated. Of course, there can be no doubt of the truth of the main incidents.

THE MISSISSIPPI PATENT FOR PULLING TEETH*

Henry Clay Lewis

Henry Clay Lewis, a graduate of a medical school, wrote as "Madison Tensas, M.D., the Louisiana Swamp Doctor." In 1850, when he was 25, his satirical sketches of medical training and practice were published as Odd Leaves from the Life of a Louisiana Swamp Doctor.—*G.P.H.F.*

I had just finished the last volume of Wistar's *Anatomy*, well nigh coming to a period myself with weariness at the same time, and with feet well braced up on the mantelpiece was lazily surveying the closed volume which lay on my lap when a hurried step in the front gallery aroused me from the revery into which I was fast sinking. Turning my head as the office door opened, my eyes fell on the well-developed proportions of a huge flat-boatman who entered the room wearing a countenance, the expression of which would seem to indicate that he had just gone into the vinegar manufacture with a fine promise of success.

"Do you pull teeth, young one?" he said to me.

"Yes, and noses, too," replied I, fingering my slender mustache, highly indignant at the juvenile appellation, and bristling up by the side of the huge Kentuckian till I looked as large as a thumb lancet by the side of an amputating knife.

"You needn't get riled, young Doc. I meant no insult, sarten, for my teeth are too sore to 'low your boots to jar them as I swallered you down. I want a tooth pulled. Can you manage the job? Ouch! criminy, but it hurts!"

"Yes, sir, I can pull your tooth. Is it an incisor, or a dens sapietiae? one of the decidua, or a permanent grinder?"

"It's a sizer, I reckon. It's the largest tooth in my jaw. Anyhow, you can see for yourself," and the Kentuckian opening the lower half of his face disclosed a set of teeth that clearly showed that his half of the alligator lay above.

"A molar requires extraction," said I, as he laid his finger on the aching fang.

"A molar! Well, I'll be cust but you doctors have queer names for things! I reckon the next time I want a money-puss a molear will be extracted too; ouch! What do you ax for pulling teeth, Doc? I want to git rid of the pesky thing."

"A dollar, sir," said I, pulling out the case of instruments and placing a chair for him.

"A dollar! dollar, h-ll! do you think the Yazoo Pass is full of kegs of speshy (specie)? I'd see you mashed under a hogshead of pork 'fore I'd give you a dollar to pull the thing," and picking up his hat, which he dashed on the floor on his first entrance, off he started.

Seeing some fun in store, I winked at the rest of the students whom the loudness of our conversation had called from the other rooms of the capacious office and requested the subject to return.

"It's no use stranger; I'd squirm all day fust 'fore I'd give you a dollar to pull every tooth in my head," said he.

"Well, Mister, times are hard, and I'll pull your tooth for half a dollar," said I, determined if necessary to give him pay before I would lose the pulling of his tooth.

"You'll have to come down a notch lower, Doc. I wants to interduce Kaintuck fashions on a Southern sile, and up thar you can get a tooth pulled and the agur 'scribed for fur a quarter."

"Well, but recollect, it's harder to pull teeth here than it is in Kentucky."

"Don't care a cuss; dimes is plentyer. I don't want to be stingy though, Doc, and I'll tell you what I'll do. I feels sorter bad from eatin' a mud cat yes-

*Reprinted with permission from Foley GPH: Dentistry and the 19th century American humorists. *New York Journal of Dentistry*, 38(9):404–406, 1968.

terday. I'll gin you a quarter to pull my tooth if you'll throw in a dose of castor ile."

"It's a bargain," said I. "I couldn't possibly afford to do it so low if I didn't manufacture my own oil and pull teeth on the 'Mississippi Patent Plan' without the least pain."

"Well, I'se struck a breeze of luck, sure, to get it 'stracted without hurtin', for I 'pected it would make all things pop, by hoecake." And "all things did pop," certain as the poor devil found to his sorrow before the "Mississippi Patent Plan" was over.

The room in which we were was the operating one of the office where patients were examined and surgical operations performed. It was furnished with all the usual appliances of such an establishment. In the middle of the room, securely fastened to the floor by screws, was a large armchair with headboard and straps to confine the body and limbs of the patient whilst the operator was at work, in such cases as required it. On either side of the house, driven into the wall, were a couple of iron bolts to which were fastened blocks and pulleys, used when reducing old dislocations when all milder means had failed. The chair, pulleys, and a small hand vise were the apparatus intended to be used by me in the extraction of the Kentuckian's tooth by the "Mississippi Patent Plan."

The patient watched all our preparations—for I quickly let the other students into the plan of the intended joke—with great interest and seemed hugely tickled at the idea of having his tooth pulled without pain for a quarter and a dose of castor oil extra.

Everything being ready, we invited the subject to take his seat in the operating chair, telling him it was necessary agreeable to our mode of pulling teeth that the body and arms should be perfectly quiet and that other doctors who hadn't bought the right to use the "Patent Plan" used the pullikins whilst I operated with the pulleys. I soon had him immovably strapped to the chair, hand and foot. Introducing the hand vise in his mouth, which fortunately for me was a large one, I screwed it fast to the offending tooth, and then connecting it with the first cord of the pulleys and intrusting it to the hands of two experienced assistants, I was ready to commence the extraction. Giving the word and singing, "Lord, receive this sinner's soul," we pulled slowly so as to let the full strain come on the neck bones gradually.

Though I live till every hair on my head is as hollow as a dry skull, I shall never forget the scene.

Clothed in homespun of the copperas hue, impotent to help himself, his body immovably fixed to the chair, his neck gradually extending itself like a terrapin's emerging from its shell, his eyes twice their natural size and projected nearly out of their sockets, his mouth widely distended with the vise hidden in its cavity, and the connection of the rope, being behind his cheeks, giving the appearance as if we had cast anchor in his stomach and were heaving it slowly home, sat the Kentuckian screaming and cursing that we were pulling his head off without moving the tooth and that the torment was awful. But I coolly told him 'twas the usual way the "Mississippi Plan" worked and directed my assistants to keep up their steady pull.

I have not yet fully determined, as it was the first and last experiment, which would have come first, his head or the tooth, for all at once the rope gave way, precipitating without much order or arrangement the assistants into the opposite corner of the room.

The operating chair, not being as securely screwed down as usual, was upturn by the shock of the retrograde motion acquired when the rope broke and landed the Kentuckian on his back in the most distant side of the room; as he fell he struck the side of his face against the wall, and out came the vise with a large tooth in its fangs. He raged like one of his indigenous thunderstorms and demanded to be released. Fearing some hostile demonstration when the straps were unfastened, we took occasion to cut them with a long bowie knife. He rose up, spitting blood and shaking himself, as if he was anxious to get rid of his clothes. "H—l, Doc, but she's a buster! I never seed such a tooth. I reckon no common fixments would have fotch it; but I tell you, sirree, it hurt awful; I think it's the last time the 'Mississippi Patent Plan' gets me in its holt. Here's a five dollar Kaintuck bill—take your pay and gin us the change."

Seeing he was in such good humor, I should have spared him, but his meanness disgusted me, and I thought I would carry the joke a little further. On examining his mouth, I suddenly discovered, as was the case, that I had pulled the wrong tooth, but I never told him, and he had too much blood in his mouth to discover it.

"Curse the luck," I exclaimed, "by Jupiter, I have lost my bet. I didn't break the infernal thing."

"Lost what?" inquired the patient, alternately spitting out blood and cramming in my tobacco.

"Why, a fine hat. I bet the old boss that the first tooth I pulled on my 'Mississippi Patent Plan' I either broke the neck of the patient or his jaw bone, and I have done neither."

"Did you ever pull a tooth that way before? Why, you told me you'd pulled a hundred."

"Yes, but they all belonged to dead men."

"And if the rope hadn't guv way, I reckon there'd bin another dead man's pulled. Cuss you, you'd never pulled my tooth if I hadn't thought you had plenty of 'sperience; but gin me my change, I wants to be gwine to the boat."

I gave the fellow his change for the five dollar bill, deducting the quarter, and the next day, when endeavoring to pass it, I found we had both made a mistake. I had pulled the wrong tooth, and he had given me a counterfeit bill.

BILL WHIFFLETREE'S DENTAL EXPERIENCE*

Jonathan F. Kelley

Jonathan F. Kelley's The Humors of Falconbridge *was published posthumously in 1856. One of these "humors" was "Bill Whiffletree's Dental Experience," a sketch depicting the suffering of the patient from unskilled treatment by a counterfeit professional.—Ed.*

Have you ever had the tooth-ache? If not, then blessed is your ignorance, for it is indeed bliss to know nothing about the tooth-ache, as you know nothing, absolutely nothing about pain—the acute, double-distilled, rectified agony that lurks about the roots or fangs of a treacherous tooth. But ask a sufferer how it feels, what it is like, how it operates, and you may learn something theoretically which you may pray heaven that you may not know practically.

But there's poor William Whiffletree—he's been through the mill, fought, bled, and died (slightly) with the refined, essential oil of the agony caused by a raging tooth. Every time we read *Othello*, we are half inclined to think that *more* than half of Iago's devilishness came from that "raging tooth," which would not let him sleep, but tortured and tormented "mine ancient" so that he became embittered against all the world, and blackamoors in particular.

William Whiffletree's case is a very strong illustration of what tooth-ache is, and what it causes people to do; and affords a pretty fair idea of the manner in which the tooth and sufferer are medicinally and morally treated by the *materia medica*, and friends at large.

William Whiffletree—or "Bill," as most people called him—was a sturdy young fellow of two-and-twenty, of "poor but respectable parents," and 'tended the dry-goods store of one Ethan Rakestraw, in the village of Rockbottom, State of New York.

One unfortunate day, for poor Bill, there came to Rockbottom a galvanized-looking individual, rejoicing in the euphonium of Dr. Hannibal Orestes Wangbanger. As a surgeon, he had—according to

the album-full of *certificates*—operated in all the scientific branches of amputation, from the scalp-lock to the heel-tap, upon Emperors, Kings, Queens, and common folks; but upon his science in the dental way, he spread and grew luminous! In short, Dr. Wangbanger had not been long in Rockbottom before his "gift of gab," and unadulterated propensity to elongate the blanket, set everybody, including poor Bill Whiffletree, in a furor to have their teeth cut, filed, scraped, rasped, reset, dug out, and burnished up!

Now Bill, being, as we aforestated, a muscularly-developed youth, got up in the most sturdy New Hampshire style, *his* teeth *were* teeth, in every way calculated to perform long and strong; but Bill was fast imbibing counter jumper notions, dabbling in stiff dickeys, greased soap locks, and other fancy "flab-dabs," supposed to be essentials in cutting a swarth among ye fair sex.

So that when Dr. Wangbanger once had an audience with Mr. William Whiffletree in regard to one of Mr. Whiffletree's molars which Bill thought had a "speck" on it, he soon convinced the victim that the said molar not only was specked, but out of the dead plum of its nearest neighbor at least the 84th part of an inch!

"O, shocking!" says the remorseless *hum*; "it is well I saw it in time, Mr. Whiffletree. Why, in the course of a few weeks, that tooth, sir, would have exfoliated, calcareous supperation would have ensued, the gum would have ossified, while the nerve of the tooth becoming apostrophized, the roots would have concatenated in their hiatuses, and the jaw-bone, no longer acting upon their fossil exoduses, would necessarily have led to the entire sus-

*Reprinted with permission from Foley GPH: Dentistry and the 19th century American humorists. *New York Journal of Dentistry*, 39(1):12–14, 19, 1969.

pension of the capillary organs of your stomach and brain, and—*death would supervene in two hours!*"

Poor Bill! he scarcely knew what fainting was, but a queer sensation settled in his "ossis frontis," while his ossis legso almost bent double under him, at the awful prospect of things before him! He took a long breath, however, and in a voice tremulous with emotion, inquired—

"Good Lord, Doctor! What's to be done for a feller?"

"Plug and file," calmly said the Doctor.

"Plug and file what?"

"The second molar," said the Doctor; though the treacherous monster *meant* Bill's wallet, of course!

"What'll it cost, Doctor?" says Bill.

"Done in my very best manner, upon the new and splendid system invented by myself, sir, and practiced upon all the crowned heads of Europe, London, and Washington City, it will cost you three dollars."

"Does it hurt much, Doctor?" was Bill's cautious inquiry.

"Very little, indeed; it's sometimes rather agreeable, sir, than otherwise," said the Doctor.

"Then go at it, Doctor! Here's the *dosh*," and forking over three dollars, down sits William Whiffletree in a highbacked chair, and the Doctor's assistant—a sturdy young Irishman—clamping Bill's head to the back of the chair, to keep it steady, as the Doctor remarked, the latter began to "bore and file."

"O! ah! ho-ho-hold on, *hold on!*" cries Bill, at the first *gouge* the Doctor gave the huge tooth.

"O—O-h-h-h!" roars Bill, as the Doctor proceeds.

"Be quiet, sir; the pain won't signify!" says the Doctor.

"Go-goo-good Lord-d-d! Ho-ho-hol-hold on!"

"O, yeez needn't be feared of that—I'm howldin yeez tight as a divil!" cried Paddy, and sure enough he *was* holding, for in vain Bill screwed and twisted and squirmed around; Pat held him like a cider-press.

"Let me—me—O—O—O! Everlasting creation! Let me go-o-o—stop, *hold on-n-n!*" as the Doctor bored, screwed, and plugged away at the tooth.

"All done, sir; let the patient up, Michael," says the Doctor, with a confident twirl of his perfumed handkerchief. "There, sir—there was science, art, elegance, and dispatch! Now, sir, your tooth is safe—your life is safe—*you're a sound man!*"

"Sound?" echoes poor Bill, "sound? Why, you've broken my jaw into flinders; you've set all my teeth on edge; and I've no more feelin'—gall darn ye!—in my jaws, than if they were iron steel-traps! You've got the wuth of your money out of my mouth, and I'm off!"

That night was one of anxiety and misery to William Whiffletree. The disturbed *molar* growled and twitched like mad; and, by daylight, poor Bill's cheek was swollen up equal to a printer's buffball, his mouth puckered, and his right eye half "bunged up."

"Why, William," says Ethan Rakestraw, as Bill went into the store, "what in grace ails thy face? Thee looks like an owl in an ivy-bush!"

"Been plugged and filed," says Bill, looking cross as a meat-axe at his snickering Orthodox boss.

"Plugged and *fined?* Thee hain't been fighting, William?"

"Fined? No I ain't been *fined* or fighting, Mr. Rakestraw, but I bet I do fight that feller who gave me the toothache!—O! O!" moaned poor Bill, as he clamped his swollen jaw with his hand, and went around waving his head like a plaster-of-paris mandarin.

"O! thee's been to the dentist, eh? Got the toothache? Go thee to my wife; she'll cure thee in one minute, William; a little laudanum and cotton will soon ease thy pain."

Mrs. Rakestraw applied the laudanum to Bill's molar, but as it did no kind of good, old grandmother proposed a poultice; and soon poor Bill's head and cheek were done up in mush, while he groaned and grunted and started for the store, everybody gaping at his swollen countenance as though he was a rare curiosity.

"Halloo, Bill!" says old Firelock, the gunsmith, as Bill was going by his shop; "got a bag in your calabash, or got the tooth-ache?"

Bill looked daggers at old Firelock, and by a nod of his head intimated the cause of his distress.

"O, that all? Come in; I'll stop it in a minute and a half; sit down, I'll fix it—I've cured hundreds," says Firelock.

"What are you—Oh-h-h, dear! What are you going to do?" says Bill, eyeing the wire, and lamp in which Firelock was heating the wire.

"Burn out the marrow of the tooth—'twill never trouble you again—I've cured hundreds that way! Don't be afeared—you won't feel it but a moment. Sit still, keep cool!" says Firelock.

"Cool?" with a hot wire in his tooth! But Bill, being already intensely crucified, and assured of Firelock's skill, took his head out of the mush-plaster, opened his jaws, and Firelock, admonishing him to "keep cool," crowded the hot, sizzling wire on to the tin foil jammed into the hollow by Wangbanger, and gave it a twist clear through the melted tin to the exposed nerve. Bill jumped, bit off the wire, burnt his tongue, and knocked Firelock nearly through the partition of his shop; and so frightened Monsieur Savon, the little barber next door, that he rushed out into the street, crying—

"Mon, Dieu! Mon Dieu! Ze zundair strike my shop!"

Bill was stone dead—Firelock crippled. The apothecary over the way came in, picked up poor Bill, applied some camphor to his nose, and brought him back to life, and—the pangs of toothache!

"Kreasote!" says Squills, the 'pothecary. "I'll ease your pain, Mr. Whiffletree, in a second!"

Poor Bill gave up—the kreasote added a fresh invoice to his misery—burnt his already lacerated and roasted tongue—and he yelled right out.

"Death and glory! O-h-h-h, murder! You've pizened me!"

"Put a hot brick to that young man's face," said a stranger; 'twill take out the pain and swelling in three minutes!"

Bill revived; he seemed pleased at the stranger's suggestion; the brick was applied; but Bill's cheek being now half raw with the various messes, it made him yell when the brick touched him!

He cleared for home, went to bed, and the excessive pain, finally, with laudanum, kreasote, fire, and hot bricks, put him to sleep.

He awoke at midnight, in a frightful state of misery; walked the floor until daylight; was tempted two or three times to jump out of the window or crawl up the chimney!

Until noon next day he suffered, trying in vain, every ten minutes, some "known cure," oils, acids, steam, poultices, and the ten thousand applications usually tried to cure a raging tooth.

Desperation made Bill revengeful. He got a club and went after Dr. Wangbanger, who had set all the village in a rage of tooth-ache. Ten or a dozen of his victims were at his door, awaiting ferociously their turns to be revenged.

But the bird had flown; the *tooth-doctor* had eloped; yet a good Samaritan came to poor Bill, and whispering in his ear, Bill started for Monsieur Savon's barber-shop, took a seat, shut his eyes, and said his prayers. The little Frenchman took a keen knife and pair of pincers, and Bill giving one awful yell, the tooth was out, and his pains and perils at an end!

BOMBASTIC BALLYHOO

The Extraordinary Advertising Life of Painless Parker*
Eric K. Curtis, D.D.S., F.A.C.D.

In 1917, San Francisco newspaper editor Fremont Older took a fancy to the flamboyant dentist Painless Parker [Edgar Randolph Parker, 1872–1952]. Parker's theatrical street pitches for outdoor dentistry had provoked a rash of malpractice suits against him in the city, as well as a sensational murder charge, and the newspapers were having a field day. But Parker claimed that the dental societies in the area, jealous of his success, were conspiring against him. Older, an anti-establishment political crusader, sympathized, and introduced Parker to local society by gaining him membership in a prestigious businessmen's group.

Sparks were bound to fly. When a well-known local dentist at one of the club's daily gatherings recognized Parker, the room went silent as he launched a verbal attack. The dentist denounced Parker as a threat to public health. "You know, Painless," the other dentist said as he raised his voice for the whole group to hear, "you really are risking your patients' lives by pulling [their] teeth on the streets. Although you may not know it, there are harmful microbes in the air. . ."

Parker was laughed out of the meeting, but he recognized an opportunity. Instead of limping home to lick his wounds, he went to a costume store and hired a man to dress up as a giant green bug. Parker walked the man back to the scene of his humiliation. "Gents," he barked, "you have just heard a learned discourse on microbes in the air from this so-called doctor. This noted scientist has told you that these germs can't be beaten by man. Well, I've gone out and brought back a bona fide microbe, and we will see if the doctor's theories hold water."

As the astonished businessmen looked on, Parker wrestled his microbe. Although he had paid the man to lose, [Parker] was beaten in two noisy bouts. "Head for the exits," Parker yelled to the crowd as the Microbe Man pinned him to the floor

for the second time. "That damn dentist was right all along!" . . .

"There is no such thing as bad publicity," media-manipulating real estate tycoon Donald Trump reportedly once said. Americans keenly sympathize with Trump's urge to be known, for, as Leo Braudy writes in his 1986 book *The Frenzy of Renown*, "We

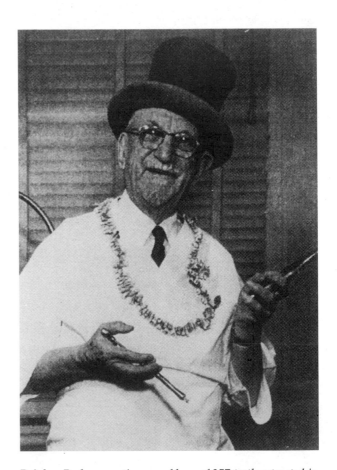

Painless Parker, sporting a necklace of 357 teeth extracted in a single day, in San Francisco shortly before his death at age 80 in 1952.

*Excerpted with permission from the *Journal of the American College of Dentists*, 62(3):55–57, 1995.

live in a society bound together by the talk of fame." Painless Parker likewise had an intuitive appreciation for the rewards of attracting attention, any kind of attention. Often posing in a top hat and a necklace made of 357 teeth he had extracted in a single day, Parker employed trumpet players, organists, mind readers, and jugglers—and for several years, even an entire circus—to gather crowds for his sales pitches. One observer described the Parker advertising approach as a spectacle of "bombastic ballyhoo."

Parker pressed the boundaries of not just respectability, but legality. He frequently called himself an "outlaw" dentist, and in many respects he was exactly that. He worked first the East Coast and then the West, sometimes practicing without a license, often staying just one step ahead of the law. When a 1915 California bill was passed prohibiting the use of an assumed name for professional purposes, Parker appeared in the San Francisco superior court and had his first name legally changed to "Painless."

Indeed, Parker's notion of professional reputation meant mostly name recognition. His trademark strategies for advertising were exaggeration and repetition. An elderly woman who had once worked for the famed dental showman was asked what she thought of Painless. "Well," she answered at length, "he wasn't."

It didn't matter to Parker that wherever he went, he stirred up storms of controversy. "When you stand up in a wagon or appear on a street corner and give a dental-hygiene sermon, some people will think you are crazy," he explained. "However, when you separate them from their cash, then who's crazy?"

Brilliantly anticipating marketing techniques that would become commonplace in other segments of American business, the relentlessly entrepreneurial Parker also franchised his operation. "You have to be organized, systematized, capitalized . . . standardized, and specialized," he advocated. "These are the major principles of business economics." Multi-state Painless Parker clinics were opened, offering a predictable appearance and standardized care, with extended hours and low fees. Parker boasted that he "brought the cost of dentistry within the reach of the masses."

The system paid off handsomely. Parker lived luxuriously, acquiring mansions, real estate, fine automobiles, and a 75-foot yacht that he sailed to Tahiti. By the early years of the 20th century Painless Parker was said to be as well-known as the president of the United States. . . .

BITS AND PIECES

COSMETIC DENTISTRY*

P. Steiner

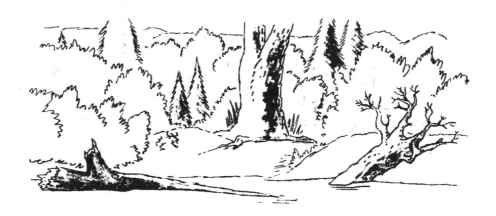

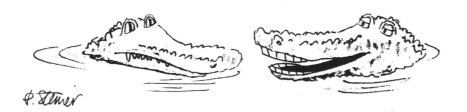

"Cosmetic dentistry changed my life."

10,000 JOKES*

One day little Flora was taken to have an aching tooth removed. That night, while she was saying her prayers, her mother was surprised to hear her say: "And forgive us our dentists as we forgive our dentists."

Dentist: I'm sorry, but I'm all out of gas."
Girl in chair: "Ye Gods! Do dentists pull that old stuff, too?"

Patient: "Do you extract teeth painlessly?"
Dentist: "Not always—the other day I nearly dislocated my wrist."

Dentist: "You needn't open your mouth any wider. When I pull your tooth I expect to stand outside."

First Cannibal: "Have you seen the dentist?"
Second Cannibal: "Yes, he filled my teeth at dinner time."

"Pardon me for a moment please," said the dentist to the victim, "but before beginning this work I must have my drill."
"Good heavens man," exclaimed the patient irritably. "Can't you pull a tooth without a rehearsal?"

Dentist (to talkative patient)—"Open your mouth and shut up."

ALWAYS UNCONSCIOUS*

One day a smart aleck got into the dentist's chair. The dentist looked at him for a moment, and then said to his attendant, "I don't dare to give him gas."
"Why not?" said the assistant.
"Because we can't tell when he loses consciousness."

*Reprinted with permission from *The Speaker's Treasury of Stories for all Occasions,* by Herbert V. Prochnow, Englewood Cliffs, NJ, Prentice Hall, Inc., 1958.

MISLAID PEARLS*

Your teeth, my love, are like the stars
That shine so bright above you;
Their pearly whiteness holds a charm
Which makes the whole world love you.
Whene'er your eyes look into mine,
They set my pulses dancing,
But when you smile at me, my love,
'Tis then you're most entrancing.
Those lovely teeth—I'll sing their praise
As long as I am able.
But do you think it proper, love,
To leave them on the table?

Anonymous

*Reprinted with permission from *10,000 Jokes, Toasts, and Stories,* by Lewis and Faye Copeland, New York, Banton-Doubleday-Dell, 1965.

*Reprinted with permission from *Dental Survey* (5)7, 1929; in *Dentistry90,* December 1990.

HUMOR VIEWS*

Swami Vichal O. Vacom was traveling in the U.S. recently when the need to visit a dentist became too great to ignore. Discovering a badly-abscessed third molar, the dentist asked what type of anesthesia the guru would prefer during the extraction.

"Oh no," answered Swami V. "That will not be necessary. Please to proceed."

"This may be quite painful," warned the dentist.

"It is all right," insisted the holy man. "I transcend dental medication."

Kit Sober

Patient: "Seventy dollars! That's an awful lot of money just to pull a tooth. It's only going to take you five minutes or so."

Dentist: "I could extract it more slowly if you'd like."

TWO GEMS OF THE DAY

Blessed are those who engage in lively conversation with the helplessly mute—for they shall be called dentists.

To keep your teeth in good condition, see your dentist twice a year and mind your own business.

Ann Landers

*Reprinted with permission by Ann Landers and Creators Syndicate.

THANKS A LOT, BUDDY*

Countryman (to dentist)—I wouldn't pay nothin' extry fer gas. Jest yank her out, if it does hurt.

Dentist—You are plucky, sir. Let me see the tooth.

Countryman—Oh, t'ain't me that's got the toothache; it's my wife. She'll be here in a minute.

*Reprinted with permission from the *California Dental Society Journal*, 23(2):14–

*Reprinted with permission from *The Bur*, 7(1), 1902; in *Dentistry 87*, April 1987.

BEWARE EXPLODING DENTURES*

The hideous charred remains of a once beautiful upper denture were sheepishly presented to me one morning by a Mr. Boswell, a baker by trade. He had bought a self-service liner from his friendly neighborhood pharmacist, taken his "impression" and, reading in the instructions that heat hastens the set, placed his denture in a warm oven for 15 minutes. He then retired to the den to watch television.

The flickering screen worked its soporific wiles: Mr. Boswell dozed off, to be precipitously awakened an hour later by the sound of "gunfire" coming from his kitchen. He rushed in and found, to his horror, that his denture had heated, softened, sagged and exploded, scattering porcelain teeth all over the oven.

But one man's loss is another man's gain, and our friendly baker had to bake a lot of brownies to pay for his new uppers!

(I was ignored by the manufacturers of home denture liners when I suggested they include the following warning on their packaging: "WARNING: THE DENTAL SURGEON GENERAL HAS DETERMINED THAT BAKING YOUR DENTURE IS HAZARDOUS TO ITS HEALTH.")

Marvin H. Leaf, D.D.S.

MARK TWAIN ON DENTISTS

When teeth became touched with decay or were otherwise ailing, the doctor knew of but one thing to do—he fetched his tongs and dragged them out. If the jaw remained, it was not his fault.

Mark Twain
From Mark Twain's Autobiography

*Reprinted with permission from the *Journal of the California Dental Association*, 23(9):16, 1995.

AUTHOR INDEX